*Step by Step*

# Corneal
# Topography

### *Editors*

**Sunita Agarwal** MS DO FSVH
Dr Agarwal's Group of Eye Hospitals
Chennai, India
and
Eye Research Centre

**Athiya Agarwal** MD DO FRSH
Dr Agarwal's Group of Eye Hospitals
Chennai, India
and
Eye Research Centre

**Amar Agarwal** MS FRCS FRC Ophth
Dr Agarwal's Group of Eye Hospitals
Chennai, India
and
Eye Research Ce

Taylor & Francis
Taylor & Francis Group

LONDON AND NEW YORK

A MARTIN DUNITZ BOOK

First published in India in 2005

**Jaypee Brothers Medical Publishers (P) Ltd, New Delhi, India.**
EMCA House, 23/23B Ansari Road, Daryaganj, New Delhi 110 002, India
Phones: 23272143, 23272703, 23282021, 23245672 m\, Fax: +91-011-23276490
e-mail: jpmedpub@del2.vsnl.net.in, Visit our website: www.jaypeebrothers.com

First published by Martin Dunitz, a member of the Taylor & Francis Group plc in 2005. Exclusively distributed worldwide (excluding the Indian Subcontinent) by Martin Dunitz, a member of the Taylor & Francis Group plc.

Tel.:      +44 (0) 1235 828600
Fax.:      +44 (0) 1235 829000
E-mail:    info@dunitz.co.uk
Website:   http://www.dunitz.co.uk

A CIP record for this book is available from the British Library.

ISBN 1 84184 547 7

Distributed in North and South America by

Taylor & Francis
2000 NW Corporate Blvd
Boca Raton, FL 33431, USA

*Within Continental USA*
Tel.: 800 272 7737; Fax.: 800 374 3401
Outside Continental USA
Tel.: 561 994 0555; Fax.: 561 361 6018
E-mail: orders@crcpress.com

Distributed in the rest of the world (excluding the Indian Subcontinent) by
Thomson Publishing Services
Cheriton House
North Way
Andover, Hampshire SP10 5BE, UK
Tel.:      +44 (0)1264 332424
E-mail:    salesorder.tandf@thomsonpublishingservices.co.uk

This book is dedicated to
A great friend,
A great surgeon,
A great teacher
and above all
A great human being.

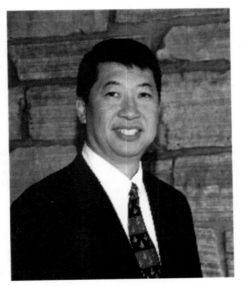

**DAVID F CHANG**

# Contributors

**Amar Agarwal** MS FRCS FRC Ophth
Consultant
Dr Agarwal's Eye Hospital
19 Cathedral Road
Chennai-600 086 (India)

**Athiya Agarwal** MD DO FRSH
Consultant
Dr Agarwal's Eye Hospital
19 Cathedral Road
Chennai-600 086 (India)
15 Eagle Street, Langford Town
Bangalore, India

**Sunita Agarwal** MS DO FSVH
Dr Agarwal's Eye Hospital
19 Cathedral Road
Chennai- 600 086 (India)
15 Eagle Street, Langford Town
Bangalore, India

**Jorge L Alió** MD
Instituto Oftalmologico De Alicante
Alicante (Spain)

**Maria C Arbelaez**
Magraby Eye Centre
AL Wattiyah, Romaila Building (106)
PO Box 513, PC 112, Rwui
Muscat, Sultanate of Oman

**Melania Cigales** MD
Instituto Oftalmologico De Sabadell
Barcelona (Spain)

**Jairo E Hoyos** MD
Instituto Oftalmologico De Sabadell
Barcelona (Spain)

**Soosan Jacob** MS FRCS
Consultant
Dr Agarwal's Eye Hospital
Chennai (India)

**Nilesh Kanjani** DO Dip NB
Dr Agarwal's Eye Hospital
Chennai, India

**Michael C Knorz**
Klinikum Mannheim
Theodor Kutzerufer 1-3
Mannheim, Germany

**Jorge Pradas**
Instituto Oftalmologico
De Sabadell
Barcelona, Spain

**José I Belda Sanchis**
Instituto Oftalmologico
De Alicante
Alicante, Spain

# Foreword

Every once in a while along comes a book that has extremely practical application, yet also presents exciting new information. Such is this *Step by Step Corneal Topography* by Drs Sunita, Athiya and Amar Agarwal that you now hold in your hands. By now, anyone who has performed 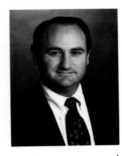 refractive surgery has struggled with reading a corneal topography map, trying to decide if it is normal or abnormal. Anyone that does cataract surgery is occasionally frustrated with a patient's postoperative outcome, wishing that the astigmatism was better addressed with the original surgery, or contemplating a second surgery to repair residual or induced astigmatism. After reviewing the contents of this corneal topography book, I am certain that you will find this difficult, often confusing mixture of science and art called corneal topography, much more manageable in your practice. Every eye care provider will come away with a new found understanding of the application of corneal topography to their practice, and will most certainly use it more often in their patient care experiences.

There are several areas of this text that are unique when compared to other texts on this subject. One is the extensive coverage of corneal topography for cataract surgery and phakonit. As lens implant surgery explodes over the next decade, and as presbyopic options for patients become more readily available, the control of astigmatism becomes critical for the excellent outcomes our patients desire and deserve. Topography is a tool that is uniquely suited for understanding the preoperative curvatures of the cornea to help plan incision site, length, construction, and suture placement if needed. The authors also have extensive coverage on not only anterior curvature based topography, which is useful, yet may give incomplete information, but this text also gives the reader insight into the importance and use of posterior corneal topography. Posterior topography uniquely applies to lens implant patients because not all patients with spherical anterior topography with refractive astigmatism have "lenticular astigmatism." Often I have been frustrated after the removal of a cataractous lens when I thought that its removal would cure the "lenticular astigmatism" in patients with refractive astigmatism, but no anterior corneal astigmatism. I was left frustrated with residual refractive astigmatism in these patients because of posterior corneal astigmatism. The author's excellent coverage of posterior corneal topography will give the reader foundation to understand the complex interaction of all refractive surfaces of the eye on their lens implant surgery, whether it is traditional forms of cataract surgery, phakic IOL surgery, or phakonit.

Also unique to this book are chapters dedicated to the topic of "Aberropia". This relatively new concept that

Drs Agarwal have helped us understand in other prior excellent textbooks, is an extremely important concept dealing with the refractive issues that are not addressed with sphere and cylinder corrections. Topography is extremely important in understanding the complex nature of what in the past we have given the rough term "irregular astigmatism." The more gentle and polished term of "aberropia" is given full life in their well written chapters. The combination of corneal topography and wavefront analysis when evaluating the refractive state of the eye can lead to correct diagnostic information in patients that then improves our ability to produce a proper spectacle, contact lens, or surgical improvement of the patient's vision and their life.

Drs Agarwal don't forget our most common use of corneal topography in this text—that of keratoconus detection. This sometimes debilitating disease of the cornea frustrates eye care providers and especially refractive surgeons to no end through its difficult diagnosis and gradual onset, with a spectrum in corneal shape from normal through severely keratoconic. Even though there is no clear cut-off as to normal versus abnormal in any disease, topography serves as a useful tool to do our best to evaluate corneas to try to predict those that may be unstable in the future. We try to predict the future course so we can try to predict the future refractive state for those patients that consult us for our opinions as to whether refractive surgery is likely to give them satisfactory results in the long term.

Drs Agarwal go the extra mile and also give the reader practical useful information on the use of topography for aberrometry guided excimer laser applications. This rapidly expanding field of customized approaches to correction of refractive states continues to grow and change, and an understanding of the concepts of topography is vital to adopt these changes in the future.

After consuming "Step by Step Series on Corneal Topography", the reader will soon realize the treasure that he or she has in their hands. This text will allow them to practice their eye care profession to the fullest, giving their patients what they really want – excellent vision.

**David R Hardten** MD FACS
Director of Refractive Surgery, Research, and
Fellowships
Minnesota Eye Consultants
Minneapolis, Minnesota
Adjunct Associate Professor of Ophthalmology
University of Minnesota
Minneapolis, Minnesota

# Preface

Ophthalmology has been making advances in leaps and bounds. It is an effort for ophthalmologists to keep abreast of every latest development.

However, a working knowledge of corneal topography has become a must, for our knowledge of the surface of the cornea was once upon a time limited to the images from the reflection of the placido's disc and that of keratometry.

Now there is a gamut of information to be obtained from the cornea and the various ways it applies to clinical ophthalmology. Even as we describe topography in detail from the basics, the reader is introduced to the Orbscan, the anterior and the lesser known posterior keratoconus.

Hence, the application of these becomes very important in preoperative and postoperative cataract and refractive surgery.

The neutrality of the phakonit incisions contrasting with the comparison of previous cataract incisions is demonstrated emphasising the need for smaller incisions on the cornea.

A startling phenomenon came to light when we studied preoperative and postoperative Aberrometer maps of LASIK patients and have termed it aberropia. We present this phenomenon called aberropia to you in this book which not only makes interesting reading but offers exciting prospects. This refractive error which is termed aberropia goes to show that we learn newer things about the eye everyday.

Last but not the least a word about LASIK assisted topography. It is the future for all LASIK and it is only a matter of time before all machines will be incorporated with an Orbscan. In this way, LASIK itself will become even more refined.

It gives us great pleasure to bring this book as it will prove to be useful to every reader.

**Sunita Agarwal**
**Athiya Agarwal**
**Amar Agarwal**

# Contents

# Chapter 1

# *Corneal Topography in Cataract Surgery*

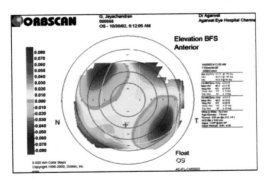

*Athiya Agarwal*
*Sunita Agarwal*
*Amar Agarwal*

## INTRODUCTION

Topography is defined as the science of describing or representing the features of a particular place in detail. In corneal topography, the place is the cornea, i.e.; we describe the features of the cornea in detail.

The word Topography is derived[1,2] from two Greek words:

TOPOS—meaning place

and

GRAPHIEN—meaning to write.

## CORNEA

There are basically three refractive elements of the eye—namely; axial length, lens and cornea. The cornea is the most important plane or tissue for refraction. This is because it has the highest refractive power (which is about + 45 D) and it is easily accessible to the surgeon without going inside the eye.

To understand the cornea, one should realize that the cornea is a parabolic curve—its radius of curvature differs from center to periphery. It is steepest in the center and flatter in the periphery. For all practical purposes the central cornea, that is the optical zone is taken into consideration, when you are doing a refractive surgery. A flatter cornea has less refraction power and a steeper cornea has a higher refraction power. If we want to change the refraction we must make the steeper diameter flatter and the flatter diameter steeper.

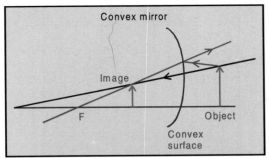

***FIGURE 1.1:*** Physics of a convex mirror. Note the image is virtual, erect and minified. The cornea acts like the convex mirror and the mire of the keratometer is the object

## KERATOMETRY

The keratometer was invented by Hermann Von Helmholtz and modified by Javal, Schiotz etc. If we place an object in front of a convex mirror we get a virtual, erect and minified image **(Figure 1.1)**. A keratometer in relation to the cornea is just like an object in front of a convex reflecting mirror. Like in a convex reflecting surface, the image is located posterior to the cornea. The cornea behaves as a convex reflecting mirror and the mires of the keratometer are the objects. The radius of curvature of the cornea's anterior surface determines the size of the image.

The keratometer projects a single mire on the cornea and the separation of the two points on the mire is used to determine corneal curvature. The zone measured depends upon corneal curvature—the steeper the cornea, the smaller the zone. For example, for a 36-D cornea, the keratometer measures a 4-mm zone and for a 50-D cornea, the size of the cone is 2.88 mm.

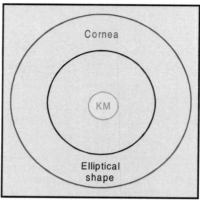

***FIGURE 1.2:*** Keratometers measure the central 3-mm of the cornea, which generally behaves like a sphere or a spherocylinder. This is the reason why keratometers are generally accurate. But in complex situations like in keratoconus or refractive surgery they become inaccurate

Keratometers are accurate only when the corneal surface is a sphere or a spherocylinder. Actually, the shape of the anterior surface of the cornea is more than a sphere or a spherocylinder. But keratometers measure the central 3-mm of the cornea, which behaves like a sphere or a spherocylinder. This is the reason why Helmholtz could manage with the keratometer **(Figure 1.2)**. This is also the reason why most ophthalmologists can manage management of cataract surgery with the keratometer. But today, with refractive surgery, the ball game has changed. This is because when the cornea has complex central curves like in keratoconus or after refractive surgery, the keratometer cannot give good results and becomes inaccurate. Thus, the advantages of the keratometer like speed, ease of use, low cost and minimum maintenance is obscured.

The objects used in the keratometer are referred to as mires. Separation of two points on the mire are used to determine corneal curvature. The object in the keratometer can be rotated with respect to the axis. The disadvantages of the keratometer are that they measure only a small region of the cornea. The peripheral regions are ignored. They also lose accuracy when measuring very steep or flat corneas. As the keratometer assumes the cornea to be symmetrical it becomes at a disadvantage if the cornea is asymmetrical as after refractive surgery.

## KERATOSCOPY

To solve the problem of keratometers, scientists worked on a system called Keratoscopy. In this, they projected a beam of concentric rings and observed them over a wide expanse of the corneal surface. But this was not enough and the next step was to move into computerized videokeratography.

## COMPUTERIZED VIDEOKERATOGRAPHY

In this some form of light like a placido disk is projected onto the cornea. The cornea modifies this light and this modification is captured by a video camera. This information is analyzed by computer software and the data is then displayed in a variety of formats. To simplify the results to an ophthalmologist, Klyce in 1988 started

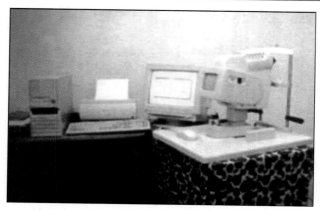

*FIGURE 1.3:* Placido type corneal topography machine

the corneal color maps. The corneal color maps display the estimate of corneal shape in a fashion that is understandable to the ophthalmologist. Each color on the map is assigned a defined range of measurement. The placido type topographic machines **(Figure 1.3)** do not assess the posterior surface of the cornea. The details of the corneal assessment can be done only with the Orbscan (Bausch and Lomb) as both anterior and posterior surface of the cornea are assessed.

## ORBSCAN

The ORBSCAN (BAUSCH & LOMB) corneal topography system **(Figure 1.4)** uses a scanning optical slit scan that is fundamentally different than the corneal topography that analyses the reflected images from the anterior corneal surface (Read Orbscan chapter 2). The high-resolution

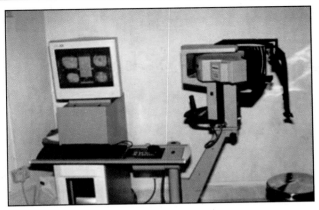

**FIGURE 1.4:** Orbscan

video camera captures 40 light slits at 45 degrees angle projected through the cornea similarly as seen during slit lamp examination. The slits are projected on to the anterior segment of the eye: the anterior cornea, the posterior cornea, the anterior iris and anterior lens. The data collected from these four surfaces are used to create a topographic map.

## NORMAL CORNEA

In a normal cornea **(Figure 1.5)**, the nasal cornea is flatter than the temporal cornea. This is similar to the curvature of the long end of an ellipse. If we see **Figure 1.5** then we will notice the values written on the right end of the pictures. These indicate the astigmatic values. In that is written Max K is 45 @ 84 degrees and Min K is 44 @ 174 degrees. This means the astigmatism is + 1.0 D at 84

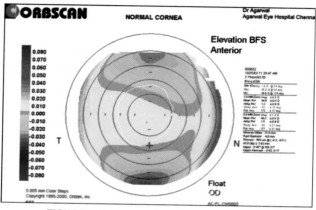

**FIGURE 1.5:** Topography of a normal cornea

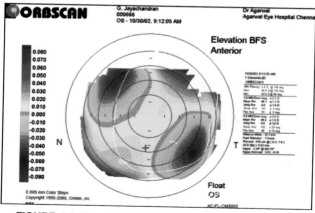

**FIGURE 1.6:** Topography showing an astigmatic cornea

degrees. This is with the rule astigmatism as the astigmatism is Plus at 90 degrees axis. If the astigmatism was Plus at 180 degrees then it is against the rule astigmatism. The normal corneal topography can be round, oval, irregular, symmetric bow tie or asymmetric bow tie in appearance. If we see **Figure 1.6** we will see a case of astigmatism in which the astigmatism is + 4.9 D at 146 degrees. *These figures show the curvature of the anterior surface of the cornea. It is important to remember that these are not the keratometric maps. So the blue/green colors denote steepening and the red colors denote flattening.* If we want the red to denote steepening then we can invert the colors.

## CATARACT SURGERY

Corneal topography is extremely important in cataract surgery. *The smaller the size of the incision lesser the astigmatism and earlier stability of the astigmatism will occur.* One can reduce the astigmatism or increase the astigmatism of a patient after cataract surgery. The simple rule to follow is that—*wherever you make an incision that area will flatten and wherever you apply sutures that area will steepen.*

### EXTRACAPSULAR CATARACT EXTRACTION

One of the problems in extracapsular cataract extraction is the astigmatism which is created as the incision size is about 10-12 mm. In **Figure 1.7**, you can see the topographic picture of a patient after extracapsular cataract extraction (ECCE). You can see the picture on the left is

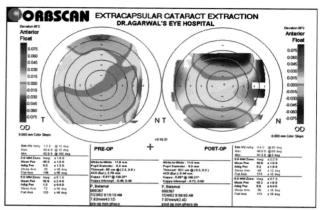

**FIGURE 1.7:** Topography after extracapsular cataract extraction (ECCE). The figure on the left shows astigmatism of + 1.1 D at 12 degrees pre-operatively. The astigmatism has increased to + 4.8 D as seen in the figure on the right

the pre-op photo and the picture on the right is a post-op day 1 photo. Pre-operatively one will notice the astigmatism is + 1.0 D at 12 degrees and post-operatively it is + 4.8 D at 93 degrees. This is the problem in ECCE. In the immediate post-operative period the astigmatism is high which would reduce with time. But the predictability of astigmatism is not there which is why smaller incision cataract surgery is more successful.

## NON-FOLDABLE IOL

Some surgeons perform phaco and implant a non-foldable IOL in which the incision is increased to 5.5 to 6 mm. In such cases the astigmatism is better than in an ECCE. In **Figure 1.8**, the pictures are of a patient who has had a

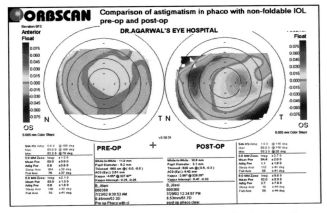

*FIGURE 1.8:* Topography of a non-foldable IOL implantation

non-foldable IOL. Notice in this the pre-operative astigmatism is + 0.8 D @ 166 degrees. This is the left eye of the patient. If we had done a phaco with a foldable IOL the astigmatism would have been nearly the same or reduced as our incision would have come in the area of the astigmatism. But in this case after a phaco a non-foldable IOL was implanted. The post-operative astigmatism one week post-op is + 1.8 D @ 115 degrees. You can notice from the two pictures the astigmatism has increased.

## FOLDABLE IOL

In phaco with a foldable IOL the amount of astigmatism created is much less than in a non-foldable IOL. Let us look now at **Figure 1.9**. The patient as you can see has negligible astigmatism in the left eye. The picture on the

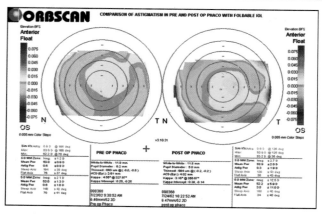

**FIGURE 1.9:** Topography of phaco cataract surgery with a foldable IOL implantation

left shows a pre-operative astigmatism of + 0.8 D at 166 degrees axis. Now, we operate generally with a temporal clear corneal approach, so in the left eye, the incision will be generally at the area of the steepend axis. This will reduce the astigmatism. If we see the post-op photo of day one we will see the astigmatism is only + 0.6 D @ 126 degrees. This means that after a day, the astigmatism has not changed much and this shows a good result. This patient had a foldable IOL implanted under the no anesthesia cataract surgical technique after a Phaco cataract surgery with the size of the incision being 2.8 mm.

## ASTIGMATISM INCREASED

If we are not careful in selecting the incision depending upon the corneal topography we can burn our hands.

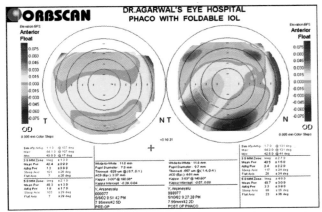

***FIGURE 1.10:*** Increase in astigmatism after cataract surgery due to incision being made in the wrong meridian. Topography of a phaco with foldable IOL implantation

**Figure 1.10**, illustrates a case in which astigmatism has increased due to the incision being made in the wrong meridian. The patient had a 2.8 mm incision with a foldable IOL implanted after a phaco cataract surgery under the no anesthesia cataract surgical technique. Both the pictures are of the right eye. In **Figure 1.10**, look at the picture on the left. In the picture on the left, you can see the patient has an astigmatism of + 1.1 D at axis 107 degrees. As this is the right eye with this astigmatism we should have made a superior incision to reduce the pre-operative astigmatism. But by mistake we made a temporal clear corneal incision. This has increased the astigmatism. Now if we wanted to flatten this case, we should have made the incision where the steeper meridian was. That was at the 105 degrees axis. But because we were doing routinely temporal clear corneal incisions, we made the incision in the opposite axis. Now look at the picture on the right. The astigmatism has increased from + 1.1 D to + 1.7 D. This shows a bad result. If we had made the incision superiorly at the 107 degrees axis, we would have flattened that axis and the astigmatism would have been reduced.

## BASIC RULE

The basic rule to follow is to look at the number written in red. The red numbers indicate the plus axis. If the difference in astigmatism is say 3 D at 180 degrees, it means the patient has + 3 D astigmatism at axis 180 degrees. This is against the rule astigmatism. In such cases, make your clear corneal incision at 180 degrees so that you can flatten this steepness. This will reduce the astigmatism.

## UNIQUE CASE

In **Figure 1.11**, the patient had a temporal clear corneal incision for Phaco cataract surgery under no anesthesia with a non-foldable IOL. Both the pictures are of the left eye. The Figure on the left shows the post-operative topographic picture. The post-operative astigmatism was + 1.8 D at axis 115 degrees. This patient had three sutures in the site of the incision. These sutures were put as a non-foldable IOL had been implanted in the eye with a clear corneal incision. When this patient came for a follow up we removed the sutures. The next day the patient

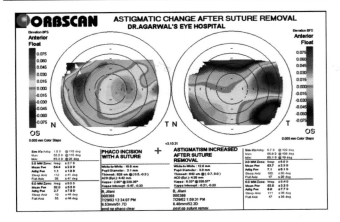

*FIGURE 1.11:* Unique case—topographic changes after suture removal

came to us with loss of vision. On examination, we found the astigmatism had increased. We then took another topography. The picture on the right is of the topography after removing the sutures. The astigmatism increased to + 5.7 D. So, one should be very careful in analyzing the corneal topography when one does suture removal also. To solve this problem one can do an astigmatic keratotomy.

## PHAKONIT

Phakonit is a technique devised by Dr.Amar Agarwal in which the cataract is removed through a 1.0 mm incision. The advantage of this is obvious. The astigmatism created by a 1.0 mm incision is very little compared to a 2.6 mm phaco incision. Today with the rollable IOL and the Acritec IOL's which are ultra-small incision IOL's one can pass IOL's

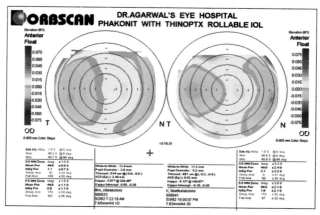

**FIGURE 1.12:** Topography of a phakonit with a rollable IOL

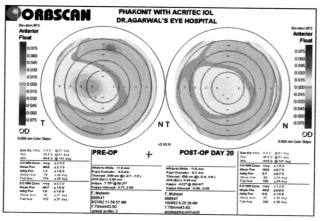

**FIGURE 1.13:** Topography of a phakonit with an acritec IOL

through sub 1.4 mm incisions. This is seen clearly in **Figures 1.12** and **1.13**. **Figure 1.12** shows the comparison after Phakonit with a Rollable IOL and **Figure 1.13** with an Acritec IOL. If you will see the pre-operative and the postoperative photographs in comparison you will see there is not much difference between the two. In this case a rollable IOL was implanted. The point which we will notice in this picture is that the difference between the pre-operative photo and the one day post-op photo is not much.

## SUMMARY

Corneal topography is an extremely important tool for the ophthalmologist. It is not only the refractive surgeon who should utilize this instrument but also the cataract surgeon. The most important refractive surgery done in the world is cataract surgery and not Lasik (Laser-in-situ keratomileusis) or PRK (Photorefractive keratectomy). With more advancements in corneal topography, Topographic- Assisted Lasik will become available to everyone with an Excimer Laser. One might also have the corneal topographic machine fixed onto the operating microscope so that one can easily reduce the astigmatism of the patient.

### REFERENCES

1. Gills JP et al. Corneal topography: The State–of-the Art. New Delhi; Jaypee Brothers Medical Publishers (P) Ltd., 1996
2. Sunita Agarwal, Athiya Agarwal, Mahipal S Sachdev, Keiki R Mehta, I Howard Fine, Amar Agarwal. Phacoemulsification, laser cataract surgery and foldable IOLs. New Delhi; Jaypee Brothers Medical Publishers (P) Ltd. 2000.

# Chapter 2

# *Orbscan*

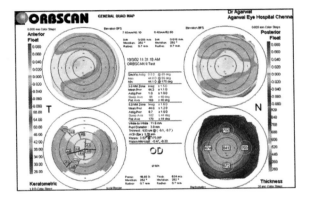

*Amar Agarwal*
*Athiya Agarwal*
*Sunita Agarwal*

# INTRODUCTION

Keratometry and corneal topography with placido discs systems were originally invented to measure anterior corneal curvature. Computer analysis of the more complete data acquired by the latter has in recent years has been increasingly more valuable in the practice of refractive surgery. The problem in the placido disc systems is that one cannot perform a slit scan topography of the cornea. This has been solved by an instrument called the Orbscan that combines both slit scan and placido images to give a very good composite picture for topographic analysis. Bausch and Lomb manufacture this.

# PARAXIAL OPTICS

Spectacle correction of sight is designed only to eliminate defocus errors and astigmatism. These are the only optical aberrations that can be handled by the simplest theory of imaging, known as paraxial optics, which excludes all light rays finitely distant from a central ray or power axis. Ignoring the majority of rays entering the pupil, paraxial optics examines only a narrow thread-like region surrounding the power axis. The shape of any smoothly rounded surface within this narrow region is always circular in cross-section. Thus from the paraxial viewpoint, surface shape is toric at most: only its radius may vary with meridional angle. As a toric optical surface has sufficient flexibility to null defocus and astigmatism, only paraxial optics is needed to specify corrective lenses for normal eyes. Paraxial optics is used in keratometers and two-dimensional topographic machines.

## RAYTRACE OR GEOMETRIC OPTICS

The initial objective of refractive surgery was to build the necessary paraxial correction in to the cornea. When outcomes are less than perfect, it is not just because defocus correction is inadequate. Typically, other aberrations (astigmatism, spherical aberration, coma, etc) are introduced by the surgery. These may be caused by decentered ablation, asymmetric healing, biomechanical response, poor surgical planning, and inadequate or misinformation. To assess the aberrations in the retinal image all the light rays entering the pupil must properly be taken in account using raytrace (or geometric) optics. Paraxial optics and its hypothetical toric surfaces must be abandoned as inadequate, which eliminates the need to measure surface curvature. Raytrace optics does not require surface curvature, but depends on elevation and especially surface slope. The Orbscan uses raytrace or geometric Optics.

## ELEVATION

Orbscan measure elevation, which is not possible in other topographic machines. Elevation is especially important because it is the only complete scalar measure of surface shape. Both slope and curvature can be mathematically derived from a single elevation map, but the converse is not necessarily true. As both slope and curvature have different values in different directions, neither can be completely represented by a single map of the surface. Thus, when characterizing the surface of non-spherical test objects used to verify instrument accuracy, elevation is always the gold standard.

Curvature maps in corneal topography (usually misnamed as power or dioptric maps) only display curvature measured in radial directions from the map center. Such a presentation is not shift-invariant, which means its values and topography change as the center of the map is shifted. In contrast, elevation is shift-invariant. An object shifted with respect to the map center is just shifted in its elevation map. In a meridional curvature view it is also described. This makes elevation maps more intuitively understood, making diagnosis easier.

To summarize:

1. Curvature is not relevant in raytrace optics.
2. Elevation is complete and can be used to derive surface curvature and slope.
3. Elevation is the standard measure of surface shape.
4. Elevation is easy to understand.

The problem we face is that there is a cost in converting elevation to curvature (or slope) and vice versa. To go from elevation to curvature requires mathematical differentiation, which accentuates the high spatial frequency components of the elevation function. As a result, random measurement error or noise in an elevation measurement is significantly multiplied in the curvature result. The inverse operation, mathematical integration used to convert curvature to elevation, accentuates low-frequency error. The Orbscan helps in good mathematical integration. This makes it easy for the ophthalmologist to understand as the machine does all the conversion.

## ORBSCAN I AND II

Previously, Orbscan I was used. This had only slit scan topographic system. Then the placido disc was added in Orbscan I. Hence Orbscan II came into the picture.

## SPECULAR VS BACK-SCATTERED REFLECTION

The keratometer eliminates the anterior curvature of the pre-corneal tear film. It is an estimate because the keratometer only acquires data within a narrow 3 mm diameter annulus. It measures the anterior tear-film because it is based on specular reflection **(Figure 2.1)**, which occurs primarily at the air-tear interface. As the keratometer has very limited data coverage, abnormal corneas can produce misleading or incorrect results.

Orbscan can calculate a variety of different surface curvatures, and on a typical eye, these are all different. Only on a properly aligned and perfectly spherical surface are the various curvatures equal. The tabulated SimK values (magnitudes and associated meridians) are the only ones designed to give keratometer- like measurements. Therefore it only makes sense to compare keratometry reading with SimK values.

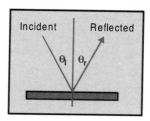

**FIGURE 2.1:** Specular reflection. This is used in keratometers. This is angle dependent

Orbscan uses slit-beams and back-scattered light **(Figure 2.2)** to triangulate surface shape. The derived mathematical surface is then raytraced using a basic keratometer model to produce simulated keratometer (SimK) values. So, it is the difficulty of calculating curvature from triangulated data, the repeatability of Orbscan I SimK values is usually not as good as a clinical keratometer. But when several readings of the same eye are averaged, no discernable systematic error is found.

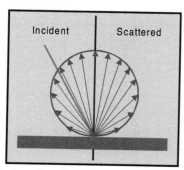

**FIGURE 2.2:** Back-scattered reflection. This is used in orbscan. This is omni-directional

So, if one reading is taken and a comparison is made, the difference may be significant enough to make you believe the instrument is not working properly. So when the placido illuminator was added to Orbscan II to increase its anterior curvature accuracy, it also provided reflected data similar to that obtained with a keratometer. This reflective data is now used in SimK analyses, resulting in repeatabilities similar to keratometers and other placido based corneal topography instruments.

Keratometry measures the tear-film, while slit-scan triangulation **(Figure 2.3)** as embodied in Orbscan sees through the tear- film and measures the corneal surface directly. Thus an abnormal tear film can produce significant differences in keratometry but not in Orbscan II.

Curvature measures the geometric bending of a surface, and its natural unit is reciprocal length, like inverse

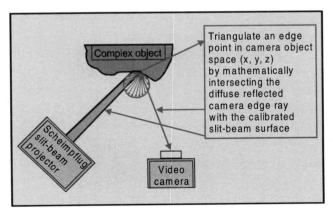

*FIGURE 2.3:* Direct triangulation

millimeters (1/mm). When keratometry was invented this unfamiliar unit was replaced by a dioptric interpretation, making keratometry values equivalent on average (i.e., over the original population) to the paraxial back-vertex power of the cornea. As it has become increasingly more important to distinguish optical from geometric properties, it is now more proper to evaluate keratometry in "keratometric diopters". The keratometric diopter is strictly defined as a geometric unit of curvature with no optical significance. One inverse millimeter equals to 337.5 keratometric diopters.

## IMAGING IN THE ORBSCAN

In the Orbscan, the calibrated slit, which falls on the cornea, gives a topographical information, which is captured and analyzed by the video camera **(Figure 2.4)**. Both slit beam surfaces are determined in camera object space. Object

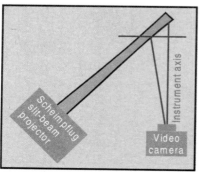

**FIGURE 2.4:** Beam and camera calibration in the orbscan

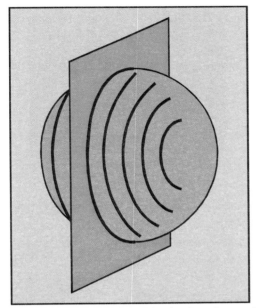

**FIGURE 2.5:** Ocular surface slicing by the orbscan slit

space luminance is determined for each pixel value and framegrabber setting. 40 Slit images are acquired in two 0.7-second periods. During acquisition, involuntary saccades typically move the eye by 50 microns. Eye movement is measured from anterior reflections of stationary slit beam and other light sources. Eye tracking data permits saccadic movements to be subtracted form the final topographic surface. Each of the 40 slit images triangulates one slice of ocular surface **(Figure 2.5)**. Before an interpolating surface is constructed, each slice is registered in accordance with measured eye movement.

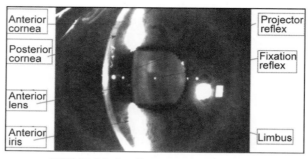

*FIGURE 2.6:* Detailed orbscan examination

Distance between data slices averages 250 microns in the coarse scan mode (40 slits limbus to limbus). So Orbscan exam consists of a set of mathematical topographic surfaces (x, y), for the anterior and posterior cornea, anterior iris and lens and backscattering coefficient of layers between the topographic surfaces (and over the pupil) **(Figure 2.6)**.

## MAP COLORS CONVENTIONS

Color contour maps have become a standard method for displaying 2-D data in corneal and anterior segment topography. Although there are no universally standardized colors, the spectral direction (from blue to red) is always organized in definite and intuitive way.

Blue = low, level, flat, deep, thick, or aberrated.

Red = high, steep, sharp, shallow, thin, or focused.

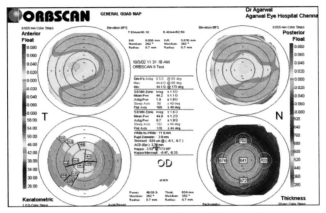

**FIGURE 2.7:** General quad map of a normal eye

## ANALYSIS OF THE NORMAL EYE BY THE ORBSCAN MAP

The general quad map in the Orbscan of a normal eye **(Figure 2.7)** shows four pictures. The upper left is the anterior float, which is the topography of the anterior surface of the cornea. The upper right shows the posterior float, which is the topography of the posterior surface of the cornea. The lower left map shows the keratometric pattern and the lower right map shows the pachymetry (thickness of the cornea). The Orbscan is a three-dimensional slit scan topographic machine. If we were doing topography with a machine, which does not have slit scan imaging facility, we would not be able to see the topography of the posterior surface of the cornea. Now, if the patient had an abnormality in the posterior surface of the cornea, for

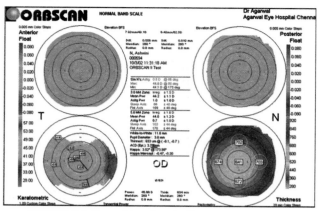

**FIGURE 2.8:** Normal band scale filter on a normal eye

example as in primary posterior corneal elevation this would not be diagnosed. Then if we perform Lasik on such a patient we would create an iatrogenic keratectasia. The Orbscan helps us to detect the abnormalities on the posterior surface of the cornea.

Another facility, which we can move onto once we have the general quad map, is to put on the normal band scale filter **(Figure 2.8)**. If we are in suspicion of any abnormality in the general quad map then we put on the normal band scale filter. This highlights the abnormal areas in the cornea in orange to red colors. The normal areas are all shown in green. This is very helpful in generalized screening in preoperative examination of a LASIK patient.

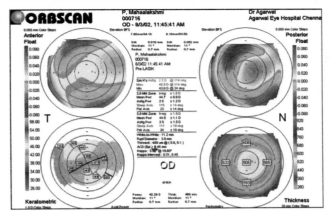

**FIGURE 2.9:** General quad map of a primary posterior corneal elevation. Notice the upper right map has an abnormality whereas the upper left map is normal. This shows the anterior surface of the cornea is normal and the problem is in the posterior surface of the cornea

## CLINICAL APPLICATIONS

Let us now understand this better in a case of a primary posterior corneal elevation. If we see the general quad map of a primary posterior corneal elevation **(Figure 2.9)** we will see the upper left map is normal. The upper right map shows abnormality highlighted in red. This indicates the abnormality in the posterior surface of the cornea. The lower left keratometric map is normal and if we see the lower right map, which is the pachymetry map one will see slightly, thin cornea of 505 microns but still one cannot diagnose the primary posterior corneal elevation only from this reading. Thus we can understand that if not for the upper right map, which denotes the posterior

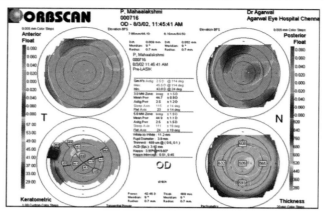

***FIGURE 2.10:*** Quad map of a primary posterior corneal elevation with the normal band scale filter on. This shows the abnormal areas in red and the normal areas are all green. Notice the abnormailty in the upper right map

surface of the cornea, one would miss this condition. The Orbscan can only diagnose this.

Now, we can put on the normal band scale filter on **(Figure 2.10)** and this will highlight the abnormal areas in red. Notice in **Figure 2.10** the upper right map shows a lot of abnormality denoting the primary posterior corneal elevation. One can also take the three-dimensional map of the posterior surface of the cornea **(Figure 2.11)** and notice the amount of elevation in respect to the normal reference sphere shown as a black grid. In a case of a keratoconus **(Figure 2.12)** all four maps show an abnormality, which confirms the diagnosis.

If we take a LASIK patients topography we can compare the pre and the post-LASIK **(Figure 2.13)**. This

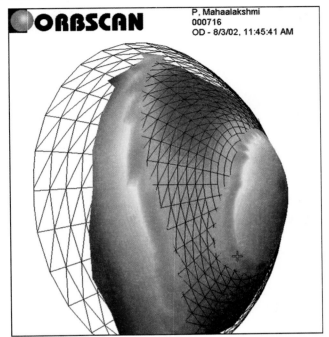

**FIGURE 2.11:** Three dimensional map of primary posterior corneal elevation. This shows a marked elevation in respect to a normal reference sphere highlighted as a black grid. Notice the red color protrusion on the black grid. This picture is of the posterior surface of the cornea

helps to understand the pattern and amount of ablation done on the cornea. The picture on the upper right is the pre-op topographic picture and the one on the lower right is the post-LASIK picture. The main picture on the left shows the difference between the pre and post-LASIK topographic patterns. One can detect from this any decentered ablations or any other complication of LASIK surgery.

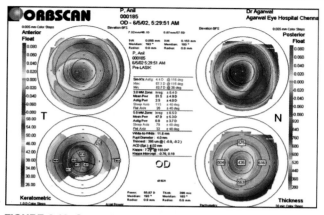

**FIGURE 2.12:** General quad map of a keratoconus patient showing abnormailty in all four maps

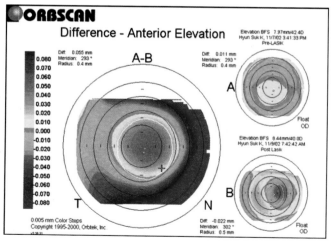

**FIGURE 2.13:** Difference of pre and post-LASIK

Corneal topography is extremely important in cataract surgery. *The smaller the size of the incision lesser the astigmatism and earlier stability of the astigmatism will occur.* One can reduce the astigmatism or increase the astigmatism of a patient after cataract surgery. The simple rule to follow is that- *wherever you make an incision that area will flatten and wherever you apply sutures that area will steepen.* One can use the Orbscan to analyze the topography before and after cataract surgery. For instance in an extracapsular cataract extraction one can check to see where the astigmatism is most and remove those sutures. In a phaco the astigmatism will be less and in Phakonit where the incision is sub 1.5 mm the astigmatism will be the least.

We can use the Orbscan to determine the anterior chamber depth and also analyze where one should place the incision when one is performing astigmatic keratotomy. The Orbscan can also help in a good fit of the contact lens with a fluorescein pattern.

## SUMMARY

The Orbscan has changed the world of topography as it gives us an understanding of a slit scan three-dimensional picture. One can use this in understanding various conditions.

# Chapter 3

# Anterior
# Keratoconus

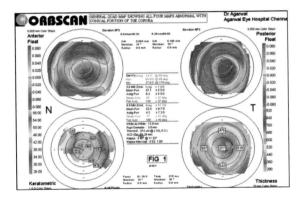

*Amar Agarwal*
*Sunita Agarwal*
*Athiya Agarwal*

## INTRODUCTION

Keratoconus is characterized by non-inflammatory stromal thinning and anterior protrusion of the cornea. Keratoconus is a slowly progressive condition often presenting in the teen or early twenties with decreased vision or visual distortion. Family history of keratoconus is seen occasionally. Patients with this disorder are poor candidates for refractive surgery because of the possibility of exacerbating keratectasia[1]. The development of corneal ectasia is a well recognized complication of LASIK and attributed to unrecognized pre-operative forme fruste Keratoconus.

## ORBSCAN

The ORBSCAN (BAUSCH & LOMB) corneal topography system uses a scanning optical slit scan that is fundamentally different than the corneal topography that analyses the reflected images from the anterior corneal surface. The high-resolution video camera captures 40 light slits at 45 degrees angle projected through the cornea similarly as seen during slit lamp examination. It has an acquisition time of 4 seconds.[2] The diagnosis of keratoconus is a clinical one and early diagnosis can be difficult on clinical examination alone. ORBSCAN has become a useful tool for evaluating the disease, and with the advent of its use, morphology and any subtle changes in the topography can be detected in early keratoconus. We always use the ORBSCAN system to evaluate our potential LASIK candidates preoperatively to rule out anterior keratoconus.

## TECHNIQUE

All eyes to undergo LASIK are examined by ORBSCAN. Eyes are screened using quad maps with the normal band (NB) filter turned on. Four maps included—(a) Anterior corneal elevation: NB = $\pm$ 25 $\mu$ of best-fit sphere. (b) Posterior corneal elevation: NB = $\pm$ 25 $\mu$ of best-fit sphere. (c) Keratometric mean curvature: NB = 40 to 48 D, K. (d) Corneal thickness (pachymetry): NB = 500 to 600 $\mu$. Map features within normal band are colored green. This effectively filters out variation falling within normal band. When abnormalities are seen on the normal band quad map screening, a standard scale quad map is examined. For those cases with anterior keratoconus, we also generate three-dimensional views of anterior and posterior corneal elevation. The following parameters are considered to detect anterior keratoconus—(a) Radii of anterior and posterior curvature of the cornea, (b) posterior best-fit sphere, (c) difference between the thickest corneal pachymetry value in 7mm zone and thinnest pachymetry value of the cornea, (d) normal band (NB) scale map, (e) elevation on the anterior float of the cornea, (f) elevation on the posterior float of the cornea, (g) location of the cone on the cornea.

## ANTERIOR KERATOCONUS

On ORBSCAN analysis in patients with anterior keratoconus the average ratio of radius of the anterior curvature to the posterior curvature of cornea is 1.25 (range 1.21 to 1.38), average posterior best-fit sphere is –56.98 Dsph (range –52.1 Dsph to –64.5), average difference in pachymetry value between thinnest point on the cornea and thickest point in 7 mm zone on the cornea is 172.7 $\mu$m (range 117 $\mu$m to 282 $\mu$m), average elevation of anterior corneal float is 55.25 $\mu$m (range 25 $\mu$m to 103 $\mu$m), average elevation of posterior corneal float is 113.6 $\mu$m (range 41 $\mu$m to 167 $\mu$m). **Figures 3.1 to 3.6** show the various topographic features of an eye with anterior keratoconus. In **Figure 3.1** (general quad map) upper left corner map is the anterior float, upper

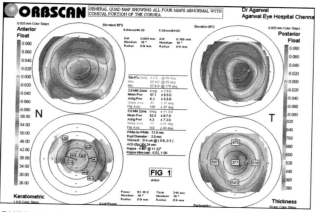

**FIGURE 3.1:** Showing general quad map of an eye with keratoconus

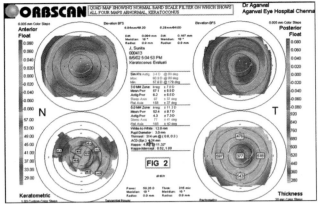

**FIGURE 3.2:** Showing quad map with normal band scale filter on in the same eye as in Figure 3.1

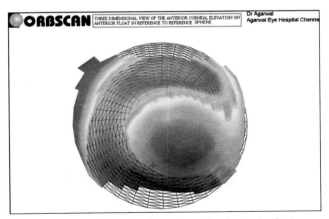

**FIGURE 3.3:** Showing three-dimensional anterior float

right corner map is posterior float, lower left corner is keratometric map while the lower right is the pachymetry map showing a difference of 282 μm between the thickest pachymetry value in 7mm zone of cornea (597 μm) and thinnest pachymetry value (315 μm). In **Figure 3.2**, normal band scale map of anterior surface shows significant elevation on the anterior and posterior float with abnormal keratometric and pachymetry maps. **Figure 3.3** is three-dimensional representation of the anterior float with reference sphere 64 μm. **Figure 3.4** shows three-dimensional representation of posterior float with reference sphere. **Figure 3.5** shows amount of elevation (color coded) of the anterior corneal surface in microns (64 μm). **Figure 3.6** shows amount of elevation (color coded) of the posterior corneal surface in microns (167 μm).

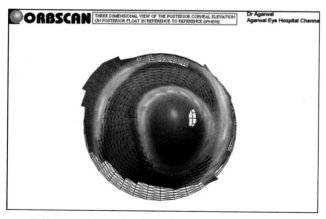

*FIGURE 3.4:* Showing three-dimensional posterior float

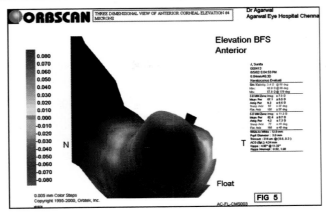

**FIGURE 3.5:** Showing three-dimensional anterior corneal elevation measured in microns

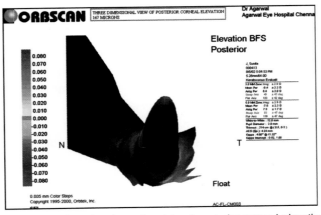

**FIGURE 3.6:** Showing three-dimensional posterior corneal elevation measured in microns

## DISCUSSION

Topography is valuable for preoperative ophthalmic examination of LASIK candidates. Three-dimensional imaging allows surgeons to look at corneal thickness, as well as the corneal anterior and posterior surface and can predict the shape of cornea after LASIK surgery. Topographic analysis using three-dimensional slit scan system allows us to predict which candidates would do well with LASIK and also confers the ability to screen for subtle configurations which may be contraindication to LASIK.[3] It is known that corneal ectasias and keratoconus have posterior corneal elevation as the earliest manifestation. In addition Wang et al have shown that the posterior corneal elevation increases after LASIK, and the increase is correlated with residual corneal bed thickness.[4] We found that patients with positive keratoconus have higher posterior and anterior elevation on Orbscan II topography.

Elevation is not measured directly by Placido based topographers, but certain assumptions allow the construction of elevation maps. Elevation of a point on the corneal surface displays the height of the point on the corneal surface relative to a spherical reference surface. Reference surface is chosen to be a sphere. Best mathematical approximation of the actual corneal surface called best-fit sphere is calculated. Posterior corneal surface topographic changes after LASIK are known. Increased negative keratometric diopters and oblate asphericity of the PCC are common after LASIK leading to mild keratectasia.[5,6] Lamellar refractive surgery reduces the biomechanical strength of cornea that may lead to mechanical instability and keratectasia. Iatrogenic keratectasia represents a complication after LASIK that may limit the range of myopic correction.[7] Corneal ectasia has also been reported after LASIK in cases of forme fruste keratoconus.[8] Posterior corneal bulge may be correlated with residual corneal bed thickness. The risk of keratectasia may be increased if the residual corneal bed is thinner than 250 $\mu$m.[9] Age, attempted correction and the optical zone diameter are other parameters that have to be considered to avoid post-LASIK ectasia.[10,11]

## CONCLUSION

The ORBSCAN provides reliable, reproducible data of the anterior corneal surface; posterior corneal surface, keratometry, and pachymetry values with three-dimensional presentations and all LASIK candidates must be evaluated by this method preoperatively to detect an " early keratoconus". We suggest that Orbscan II is an important pre-operative investigative tool to decide the suitable candidate for LASIK and thus avoiding any complication of LASIK surgery and helping the patient out by contact lens or keratoplasty. The following parameters must be analyzed in all LASIK candidates to rule out keratoconus—(a) ratio of radii of anterior to posterior curvature of cornea: > 1.21 and < 1.27 (b) posterior best fit sphere: > –52.0 Dsph (c) difference between thickest corneal pachymetry value at 7mm zone and thinnest pachymetry value: > 100 $\mu$m, (d) posterior corneal elevation > 50 $\mu$m.

## REFERENCES

1. Seiler T, Quurke AW. Iatrogenic keratectasia after LASIK in a case of forme fruste keratoconus. J Cataract Refract Surg 1998;24:1007-09.
2. Fedor P, Kaufman S Corneal topography and imaging. Medicine Journal, 2001;vol 2, no 6.
3. McDermott G K Topography's benefits for LASIK. Review of Ophthalmology. Editorial, vol no: 9:03 issue.
4. Wang Z, Chen J, Yang B. Posterior corneal surface topographic changes after laser in situ keratomileusis are related to residual corneal bed thickness. Ophthalmology 1999; 106: 406-9; discussion 409-10.
5. Seitz B, Torres F, Langenbucher A, et al. Posterior corneal curvature changes after myopic laser in situ keratomileusis. Ophthalmology 2001 April; 108 (4): 666-72.
6. Geggel H S, Talley A R. Delayed onset keratectasia following laser in situ keratomileusis. J Cataract Refract Surg 1999 Apr; 25(4): 582-86.
7. Seiler T, Koufala K, Richter G. Iatrogenic keratectasia after laser in situ keratomileusis. J Refract Surg 1998 May-June; 14(3): 312-17.
8. Seiler T, Quurke A W. Iatrogenic keratectasia after laser in situ keratomileusis in a case of Forme Fruste keratoconus. J Refract Surg 1998 Jul;24(7): 1007-09.
9. Wang Z, Chen J, Yang B. Posterior corneal surface topographic changes after laser in situ keratomileusis are related to residual corneal bed thickness. Ophthalmology 1999 Feb; 106(2): 406-09.
10. Pallikaris I G, Kymionis G D. Astyrakakis N I. Corneal ectasia induced by laser in situ keratomileusis. J Cataract Refract Surg 2001 Nov; 27(11): 1796-802.
11. Argento C, Cosentino M J, Tytium A et al. Corneal ectasia after laser in situ keratomileusis. J Cataract Refract Surg 2001 Sep; 27(9): 1440-810.

# Chapter 4

# Posterior Corneal Changes in Refractive Surgery

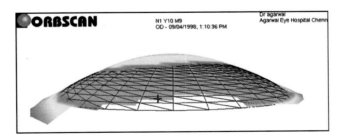

*Amar Agarwal*
*Soosan Jacob*
*Sunita Agarwal*
*Athiya Agarwal*
*Nilesh Kanjani*

## INTRODUCTION

The development of corneal ectasia is a well-recognized complication of LASIK and amongst other contributory factors, unrecognized pre-operative forme fruste keratoconus is also an important one. Patients with this disorder are poor candidates for refractive surgery because of the possibility of exacerbating keratectasia. It is known that posterior corneal elevation is an early presenting sign in keratoconus and hence *it is imperative to evaluate posterior corneal curvature (PCC) in every LASIK candidate.*

## TOPOGRAPHY

Topography is valuable for preoperative ophthalmic examination of LASIK candidates. Three-dimensional imaging allows surgeons to look at corneal thickness, as well as the corneal anterior and posterior surface and it can also predict the shape of the cornea after LASIK surgery. Topographic analysis using three-dimensional slit scan system allows us to predict which candidates would do well with LASIK and also confers the ability to screen for subtle configurations which may be a contraindication to LASIK.

## ORBSCAN

*The ORBSCAN (BAUSCH & LOMB) corneal topography system uses a scanning optical slit scan which makes it fundamentally different from the corneal topography that analyses the reflected images from the anterior corneal surface.* The high-resolution video camera captures 40 light slits at 45 degrees angle projected through the cornea similarly as seen during slit lamp examination. The slits are projected on to the anterior segment of the eye: the anterior cornea, the posterior cornea, the anterior iris and anterior lens. The data collected from these four surfaces are used to create a topographic map. Each surface point from the diffusely reflected slit beams that over-lap in the central 5-mm zone is independently triangulated to x, y, and z coordinates, providing three-dimensional data.

This technique provides more information about the anterior segment of the eye, such as anterior and posterior corneal curvature, elevation maps of the anterior and posterior corneal surface and corneal thickness. It has an acquisition time of 4 seconds.[1] This improves the diagnostic accuracy. It also has passive eye-tracker from frame to frame and 43 frames are taken to ensure accuracy. It is easy to interpret and has good repeatability.

## PRIMARY POSTERIOR CORNEAL ELEVATION

The diagnosis of frank keratoconus is a clinical one. Early diagnosis of forme fruste can be difficult on clinical examination alone. ORBSCAN has become a useful tool for evaluating the disease, and with its advent, abnormalities in posterior corneal surface topography have been identified in keratoconus. Posterior corneal surface data is problematic because it is not a direct measure and there is little published information on normal values for each age group. In the patient with increased posterior corneal elevation in the absence of other changes, it is unknown whether this finding represents a manifestation of early keratoconus. The decision to proceed with refractive surgery is therefore more difficult.

## POSTERIOR CORNEAL TOPOGRAPHY

One should always use the ORBSCAN system to evaluate potential LASIK candidates preoperatively to rule out primary posterior corneal elevations. Eyes are screened using quad maps with the normal band (NB) filter turned on. Four maps include (a) anterior corneal elevation: NB $= \pm 25 \mu$ of best-fit sphere. (b) posterior corneal elevation: NB $= \pm 25 \mu$ of best fit sphere. (c) Keratometric mean curvature: NB = 40 to 48 D (d) Corneal thickness (pachymetry): NB = 500 to 600 $\mu$. Map features within normal band are colored green. This effectively filters out variations falling within the normal band. When abnormalities are seen on normal band quad map screening, a standard scale quad map should be examined. For those cases with posterior corneal elevation, three-dimensional views of posterior corneal elevation can also be generated. In all eyes with posterior corneal elevation, the following parameters are generated (a) radii of anterior and posterior curvature of the cornea, (b) posterior best fit sphere, (c) difference between the corneal pachymetry value in 7mm zone and thinnest pachymetry value of the cornea.

## PREEXISTING POSTERIOR CORNEAL ABNORMALITIES

**Figures 4.1 to 4.6** show the various topographic features of an *eye* with primary posterior corneal elevation detected during pre-LASIK assessment. In **Figure 4.1** (general quad map) upper left corner map is the anterior float, upper right corner map is posterior float, lower left corner is keratometric map while the lower right is the pachymetry map showing a difference of 100 μm between the thickest pachymetry value in 7mm zone of cornea and thinnest pachymetry value. In **Figure 4.2**, normal band scale map of anterior surface shows "with the rule astigmatism" in an otherwise normal anterior surface (shown in green), the posterior float shows significant elevation inferotemporally. In **Figure 4.2** only the abnormal areas are shown in red for ease in detection. **Figure 4.3** is three-dimensional representation of the maps in **Figure 4.2**. **Figure 4.4** shows three-dimensional representation of anterior corneal surface with reference sphere. **Figure 4.5** shows three-dimensional representation of posterior corneal surface showing a significant posterior corneal elevation. **Figure 4.6** shows amount of elevation (color coded) of the posterior corneal surface in microns (50 μm).

In the light of the fact that keratoconus may have posterior corneal elevation as the earliest manifestation, preoperative analysis of posterior corneal curvature to detect a posterior corneal bulge is important to avoid post LASIK keratectasia. The rate of progression of posterior

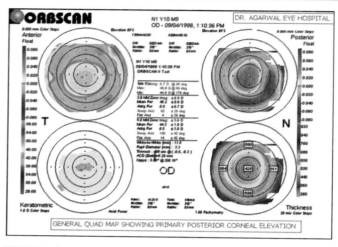

**FIGURE 4.1:** Showing general quad map of an eye with primary posterior corneal elevation. Notice the red areas seen in the top right picture showing the primary posterior corneal elevation

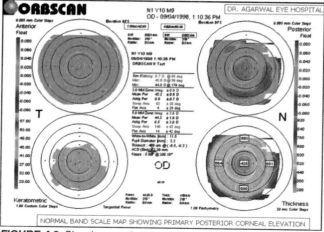

**FIGURE 4.2:** Showing quad map with normal band scale filter on in the same eye as in Figure 4.1

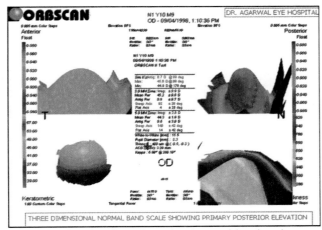

THREE DIMENSIONAL NORMAL BAND SCALE SHOWING PRIMARY POSTERIOR ELEVATION

***FIGURE 4.3:*** Showing three-dimensional normal band scale map. In the top right. Note the red areas which shows the elevation on the posterior cornea. The anterior cornea is normal.

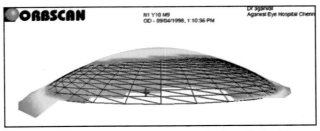

***FIGURE 4.4:*** Showing three-dimensional anterior float. Notice it is normal

corneal elevation to frank keratoconus is unknown. It is also difficult to specify that exact amount of posterior corneal elevation beyond which it may be unsafe to carry out LASIK. Atypical elevation in the posterior corneal map more than 45 $\mu$m should alert us against a post LASIK surprise. ORBSCAN provides reliable, reproducible data

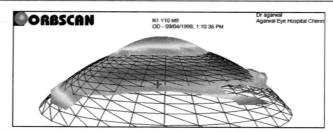

**FIGURE 4.5:** Showing three-dimensional posterior float. Notice in this there is marked elevation as seen in the red areas

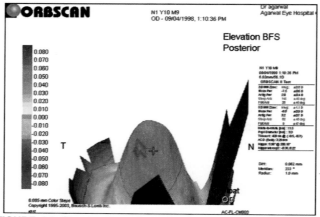

**FIGURE 4.6:** Showing three-dimensional posterior corneal elevation measured in microns

of the posterior corneal surface and all LASIK candidates must be evaluated by this method preoperatively to detect an " early keratoconus".

Elevation is not measured directly by Placido based topographers, but certain assumptions allow the construction of elevation maps. Elevation of a point on the corneal surface displays the height of the point on the corneal surface relative to a spherical reference surface. Reference surface is chosen to be a sphere. Best mathematical approximation of the actual corneal surface called best-fit sphere is calculated. One of the criteria for defining forme fruste keratoconus is a posterior best fit sphere of > 55.0 D.

Ratio of radii of anterior to posterior curvature of cornea ³ 1.21 and £ 1.27 has been considered as a keratoconus suspect. Average pachymetry difference between thickest and the thinnest point on the cornea in the 7 mm zone should normally be less than 100 $\mu$m.

## AGARWAL CRITERIA TO DIAGNOSE PRIMARY POSTERIOR CORNEAL ELEVATION

1. Ratio of the Radii of anterior and posterior curvature of the cornea should be more than 1.2. In **Figure 4.2** note the radii of the anterior curvature is 7.86 mm and the radii of the posterior curvature is 6.02 mm. The ratio is 1.3.
2. Posterior best fit sphere should be more than 52 D. In **Figure 4.2** note the posterior best fit sphere is 56.1 D
3. Difference between the thickest and thinnest corneal pachymetry value in the 7 mm zone should be more than 100 microns. The thickest pachymetry value as seen in Figure 4.2 is 651 microns and the thinnest value is 409 microns. The difference is 242 microns
4. The thinnest point on the cornea should correspond with the highest point of elevation of the posterior corneal surface. The thinnest point as seen in Figure

4.2 bottom right picture is seen as a cross. This point or cursor corresponds to the same cross or cursor in **Figure 4.2** top right picture which indicates the highest point of elevation on the posterior cornea.

5. Elevation of the posterior corneal surface should be more than 45 microns above the posterior best fit sphere. In **Figure 4.2** you will notice it is 0.062 mm or 62 microns.

## IATROGENIC KERATECTASIA

Iatrogenic keratectasia may be seen in some patients following ablative refractive surgery **(Figures 4.7 and 4.8)**. The anterior cornea is composed of alternating collagen fibrils and has a more complicated interwoven structure than the deeper stroma and it acts as the major stress-bearing layer. The flap used for LASIK is made in this layer and thus results in a weakening of that strongest layer of the cornea which contributes maximum to the biomechanical stability of the cornea.

*The residual bed thickness (RBT) of the cornea is the crucial factor contributing to the biomechanical stability of the cornea after LASIK.* The flap as such does not contribute much after its repositioning to the stromal bed. This is easily seen by the fact that the flap can be easily lifted up even up to 1 year after treatment. The decreased RBT as well as the lamellar cut in the cornea both contribute to the decreased biomechanical stability of the cornea. A reduction in the RBT results in a long term increase in the

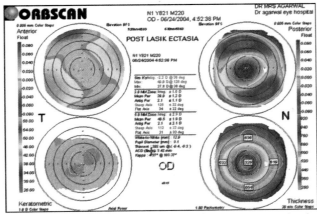

**FIGURE 4.7:** Shows a patient with iatrogenic keratectasia after lasik. Note the upper right hand corner pictures showing the posterior float has thinning and this is also seen in the bottom right picture in which pachymetry reading is 329

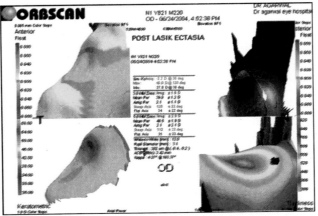

**FIGURE 4.8:** Shows the same patient with iatrogenic keratectasia after lasik in a 3 D pattern. Notice the ectasia seen clearly in the bottom right picture

surface parallel stress on the cornea. The intraocular pressure (IOP) can cause further forward bowing and thinning of a structurally compromised cornea. Inadvertent excessive eye rubbing, prone position sleeping, and the normal wear and tear of the cornea may also play a role. The RBT should not be less than 250 mm to avoid subsequent iatrogenic keratectasias. [2-4] Reoperations should be undertaken very carefully in corneae with RBT less than 300 mm. Increasing myopia after every operation is known as "dandelion keratectasia".

*The ablation diameter also plays a very important role in LASIK.* Post-operative optical distortions are more common with diameters less than 5.5 mm. Use of larger ablation diameters implies a lesser RBT post-operatively. Considering the formula: Ablation depth [mm] = 1/3. diameter [mm])$^2$ x (intended correction diopters [D]),[4,5] it becomes clear that to preserve a sufficient bed thickness, the range of myopic correction is limited and the upper limit of possible myopic correction may be around 12 D.[6]

Detection of a mild keratectasia requires knowledge about the posterior curvature of the cornea. Posterior corneal surface topographic changes after LASIK are known. Increased negative keratometric diopters and oblate asphericity of the PCC, which correlate significantly with the intended correction are common after LASIK leading to mild keratectasia.[6,7] This change in posterior power and the risk of keratectasia was more significant with a RBT of 250 $\mu$m or less.[8] The difference in the refractive indices results in a 0.2 D difference at the back surface of the cornea becoming equivalent to a 2.0 D change in the front surface of the cornea.[6] Increase in posterior power and asphericity also correlates with the difference between the intended and achieved correction 3 months after LASIK. This is because factors like drying of the stromal bed may result in an ablation depth more than that intended.[6] Reinstein et al predict that the standard deviation of uncertainty in predicting the RBT preoperatively is around 30 $\mu$m. [Invest Ophthalmol Vis Sci 40 (Suppl):S403, 1999]. Age, attempted correction, the optical zone diameter and the flap thickness are other parameters that have to be considered to avoid post LASIK ectasia.[9,10]

The flap thickness may not be uniform throughout its length. In studies by Seitz et al, it has been shown that the Moris Model One microkeratome and the Supratome cut deeper towards the hinge, whereas the Automated Corneal Shaper and the Hansatome create flaps that are thinner towards the hinge. Thus, accordingly, the area of corneal ectasia may not be in the centre but paracentral, especially if it is also associated with decentered ablation. Flap thickness has also been found to vary considerably, even upto 40 $\mu$m, under similar conditions and this may also result in a lesser RBT than intended.[11-17]

It is known that corneal ectasias and keratoconus have posterior corneal elevation as the earliest manifestation.[18] The precise course of progression of posterior corneal elevation to frank keratoconus is not known. Hence it is necessary to study the posterior corneal surface preoperatively in all LASIK candidates.

## EFFECT OF POSTERIOR CORNEAL CHANGE ON IOL CALCULATION

IOL power calculation in post-LASIK eyes is different because of the inaccuracy of keratometry, change in anterior and posterior corneal curvatures, altered relation between the two and change in the standardized index of refraction of the cornea. Irregular astigmatism induced by the procedure, decentered ablations and central islands also add to the problem.

Routine keratometry is not accurate in these patients. Corneal refractive surgery changes the asphericity of the cornea and also produces a wide range of powers in the central 5mm zone of the cornea. *LASIK makes the cornea of a myope more oblate so that keratometry values may be taken from the more peripheral steeper area of the cornea, which results in calculation of a lower than required IOL power resulting in a hyperopic "surprise". Hyperopic LASIK makes the cornea more prolate, thus resulting in a myopic "surprise" post-cataract surgery.*

Post PRK or LASIK, the relation between the anterior and posterior corneal surface changes. The relative thickness of the various corneal layers, each having a different refractive index also changes and there is a change in the curvature of the posterior corneal surface. All these result in the standardized refractive index of 1.3375 no longer being accurate in these eyes.

At present there is no keratometry, which can accurately measure the anterior and posterior curvatures of the cornea. The Orbscan also makes mathematical assumptions of the posterior surface rather than direct measurements. This is important in the LASIK patient because the procedure alters the relation between the anterior and posterior surfaces of the cornea as well as changes the curvature of the posterior cornea.

Thus direct measurements such as manual and automated keratometry and topography are inherently inaccurate in these patients. The corneal power is therefore calculated by the calculation method, the contact lens overrefraction method and by the CVK method. The flattest K reading obtained by any method is taken for IOL power calculation (the steepest K is taken for hyperopes who had undergone LASIK). One can still aim for 1.00 D of myopia rather than emmetropia to allow for any error, which is almost always in the hyperopic direction in case of pre LASIK myopes. Also, a third or fourth generation IOL calculating formula should be used for such patients.

# REFERENCES

1. Fedor P, Kaufman S. Corneal topography and imaging. Medicine Journal, 2001; 2(6).
2. Seiler T, Koufala K, Richter G. Iatrogenic keratectasia after laser in situ keratomileusis. J Refract Surg 1998;14(3):312-17.
3. Seiler T, Quurke A W. Iatrogenic keratectasia after laser in situ keratomileusis in a case of Forme Fruste keratoconus. J Refract Surg 1998;24(7):1007-09.

4. Probost LE, Machat JJ. Mathematics of laser in situ keratomileusis for high myopia. J Cataract refract Surg 1998;24.

5. Mc Donnell PJ. Excimer laser corneal surgery: new strategies and old enemies {review}. Invest Ophthalmol Vis Sci 1995; 36;4-8.

6. Seitz B, Torres F, Langenbucher A, et al. Posterior corneal curvature changes after myopic laser in situ keratomileusis. Ophthalmology 2001;108 (4): 666-72.

7. Geggel H S, Talley A R. Delayed onset keratectasia following laser in situ keratomileusis. J Cataract Refract Surg 1999; 25(4):582-86.

8. Wang Z, Chen J, Yang B. Posterior corneal surface topographic changes after laser in situ keratomileusis are related to residual corneal bed thickness. Ophthalmology 1999;106(2):406-09.

9. Pallikaris I G, Kymionis G D. Astyrakakis N I. Corneal ectasia induced by laser in situ keratomileusis. J Cataract Refract Surg 2001;27(11):1796-802.

10. Argento C, Cosentino M J, Tytium A et al. Corneal ectasia after laser in situ keratomileusis. J Cataract Refract Surg 2001; 27(9): 1440-48.

11. Binder PS, Moore M. Lambert RW et al. Comparison of two microkeratome systems. J refract surg; 1997;13;142-53.

12. Hofmann RF, Bechara SJ. An independent evaluation of second generation suction microkeratomes. Refract Corneal Surg 1992;8:348-54.

13. Schuler A, Jessen K, Hoffmann F. accuracy of the microkeratome keratectomies in pig eyes. Invest Ophthalmol Vis Sci 1990;31:2022-30.

14. Behrens A, Seitz B, Langenbucher A et al. Evaluation of corneal flap dimensions and cut quality using a manually guided microkeratome [published erratum appears in J Refract Surg 1999;15:400]. J Refract Surg 1999;15:118-23.

15. Behrens A, Seitz B, Langenbucher A et al. Evaluation of corneal flap dimensions and cut quality using the Automated Corneal Shaper microkeratome. J Refract Surg 2000;16:83-9.

16. Behrens A, Langenbucher A, Kus MM, et al. Experimental evaluation of two current generation automated micro-keratomes: the Hansatome® and the Supratome®. Am J Ophthalmol 2000;129:59-67.
17. Jacobs BJ, Deutsch TA, Rubenstein JB. Reproducibility of corneal flap thickness in LASIK. Ophthalmic Surg Lasers 1999;30:350-53.
18. McDermott G K Topography's benefits for LASIK. Review of Ophthalmology. Editorial, vol no:9:03 issue.

# Chapter 5

# *Irregular Astigmatism: Diagnosis and Management*

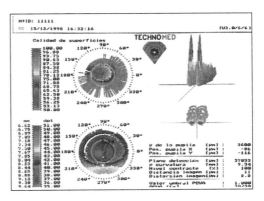

*Jorge L Alió*
*José I Belda Sanchis*

## INTRODUCTION

Irregular astigmatism is one of the most difficult and frustrating problems in refractive surgery and one of the worst sequels of corneal injuries. With the recent evolution of refractive surgery, new types of irregular astigmatism are being observed.

The astigmatism is defined as irregular if the principal meridians are not 90 degrees apart, usually because of an irregularity of the corneal curvature. It cannot be completely corrected with a sphero-cylindrical lens.[1] The alternatives for correction of irregular astigmatism are very scarce and with very limited expectations. Spectacle correction is usually not useful in the correction of corneal irregular astigmatism. Contact lens are a good alternative, but its adaptation and stability is limited by irregularity corneal surface and the patient's comfort. We must also remember that our patients are need to be consented for refractive surgery because they do not want to use contact lens any more.

Lamellar graft and fullthickness corneal grafting are surgical alternatives that are happened in practice by limited availability of corneal donor as well as by the biological and refractive complications of allografic corneal graft. Many surgeons have made great efforts in finding a solution to this problem.[2-4] Till this date, we believe there are safe, efficient and predictable methods to resolve this problem. For all these reasons, the approach to new surgical methods for the correction of irregular astigmatism is one of the biggest expectations in today's refractive surgery, specially when the generalization of corneal refractive surgical technique is to be expected in the immediate future.

## CLINICAL CLASSIFICATION OF IRREGULAR ASTIGMATISM

In corneal refractive surgery using laser *in situ* keratomileusis (LASIK) the surgeons use an automated or manual microkeratome for the creation of the corneal flap and stromal bed. Once the flap is made, the excimer laser is used to ablate tissue from the bed for the planned correction, depending on the capabilities of the laser.

From a clinical point of view, irregular astigmatism induced by LASIK can be classified as:

1. **Superficial:** If astigmatism is due to flap irregularities.
2. **Stromal:** If astigmatism is induced by bed irregularities.
3. **Mixed:** When astigmatism is due to irregularities in both flap and stroma.

## CORNEAL TOPOGRAPHY PATTERNS OF IRREGULAR ASTIGMATISM

The classification of topography patterns is very important for the following reasons:

1. To unify terms and concepts when we refer to images of corneal topography.
2. To determine the cause of the subjective symptoms, referred by the patient. Spherical and optical aberrations: Haloes, glare, monocular diplopia, etc.

3. To establish a topographic basis for a new treatment. For these patients with a previous unsuccessful excimer laser treatment, a topographic approach for treatment would allow surgeons to reshape the cornea in any pattern they choose.

We divide irregular astigmatism in two groups:
1. Irregular astigmatism with defined pattern
2. Irregular astigmatism with undefined pattern.

## IRREGULAR ASTIGMATISM WITH DEFINED PATTERN

We define irregular astigmatism with defined pattern when there is a steep or flat area of at least 2 mm of diameter, at any location of the corneal topography, which is the main cause of the irregular astigmatism. It is divided into five groups:

### Decentered Ablation

It shows a corneal topographic pattern with decentered myopic ablation in more than 1.5 mm in relation to the center of the cornea. The flattening area is not centered in the center of the cornea, the optical zone of the cornea has one flat and one steep area **(Figure 5.1)**.

### Decentered Steep

It shows a corneal hyperopic treatment decentered in more than 1.5 mm in relation to the center of the cornea **(Figure 5.2)**.

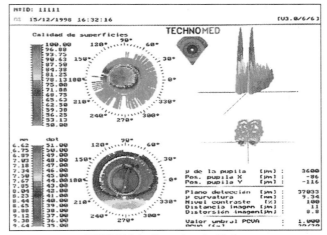

**FIGURE 5.1:** Decentered ablation

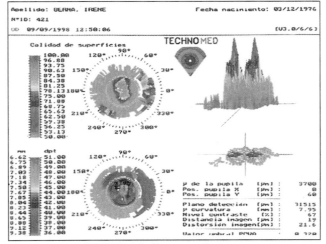

**FIGURE 5.2:** Decentered steep

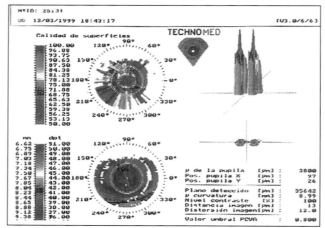

**FIGURE 5.3:** Central island

### Central Island

It shows an image with an increase in the central power of the ablation zone for myopic treatment ablation at least 3.00 D and 1.5 mm in diameter, surrounded by areas of lesser curvature **(Figure 5.3)**.

### Central Irregularity

It shows an irregular pattern with more than one area not larger than 1.0 mm and no more than 1.50 D in relationship with the flattest radius, located into the area of the myopic ablation treatment **(Figure 5.4)**.

### Peripheral Irregularity

It is a corneal topographic pattern, similar to central island, extending to the periphery. The myopic ablation is not

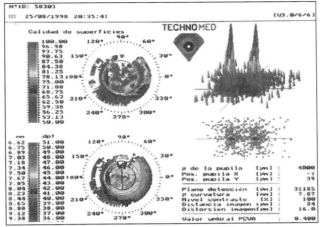

**FIGURE 5.4:** Central irregularity

homogeneous, there is a central zone measuring 1.5 mm in diameter and 3.00 D in relation to the flattest radius, connected with the periphery of the ablation zone in one meridian **(Figure 5.5)**.

## IRREGULAR ASTIGMATISM WITH UNDEFINED PATTERN (IRREGULARLY IRREGULAR)

We consider irregular astigmatism with undefined pattern when the image shows a surface with multiples irregularities; big and small steep and flat areas, defined as more than one area measuring more than 3 mm in diameter in the central 6 mm **(Figure 5.6)**. The difference between flat and steep areas were not possible to calculate in the Profile Map and Dk showed an irregular line or a plane line. Normally, Dk is the difference between the steep k

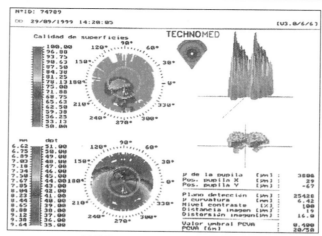

**FIGURE 5.5:** Peripheral irregularity

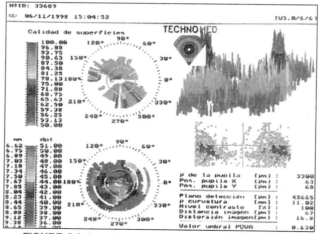

**FIGURE 5.6:** Irregular astigmatism with undefined pattern
(irregularly irregular)

and the flat k, given in diopters at the cross of the profile map. A plane line is produced when the Dk cannot recognize the difference between the steep k and the flat k in severe corneal surface irregularities.

## EVALUATION OF IRREGULAR ASTIGMATISM

A complete preoperative ocular examination was performed, including previous medical reports and complete ocular examination: uncorrected and best-corrected visual acuity, pinhole visual acuity and cycloplegic refraction, keratometry, contact ultrasonic pachymetry (Ophthasonic Pachymeter Teknar Inc. St. Louis, USA) and computerized corneal topography. We performed corneal topography with Eye Sys 2000 Corneal Analysis System (Eye Sys Co., Houston, Texas, USA). We also used the C-SCAN Color-Ellipsoid-Topometer (Technomed GmbH, Germany) to determine the Superficial Corneal Surface Quality (SCSQ) and the Predicted Corneal Visual Acuity (PCVA), using the Ray Tracing mode. Recently, we have incorporated the elevation topography (Orbtek, Bausch and Lomb Surgical, Orbscan II corneal topography, Salt Lake City, Utah). Follow up examinations after surgery were performed at 48 hours, and then at one, three and six months. Postoperative follow up included: uncorrected and best-corrected visual acuity, pinhole visual acuity and cycloplegic refraction, biomicroscopy with slit lamp and complete corneal topography screening with the previously mentioned instrumentation.

During the preoperative and postoperative period, the surface quality of the cornea was studied using the Ray Tracing module of the C-SCAN 3.0 (Technomed GmbH, Germany). This device determines the Predicted Corneal Visual Acuity from the videokeratography map, by simulating the propagation of rays emanating from 2 light dots, which impinge on the best-fit image plane after projection via the maximum of 10,800 previously determined corneal surface power values. Refraction and reflection of the rays at the optical interfaces, the pupil diameter, and the anterior chamber depth are taken into account according to laws of geometric optics. The Ray Tracing module calculates the pupil size by the captured image of the pupil during videokeratography. This is measured under the luminance of the videokeratography rings ($25.5$ cd/m$^2$) and is automatically integrated into the Ray Tracing analysis with the videokeratography map. Hence, the projection of objects onto a detection plane can be determined. The Ray Tracing module calculates the optical function of the eye by means of optical Ray Tracing, using the cornea as the refractive element of the system. It measured and analyzed the interaction between the corneal shape, the functional optical zone, and the pupil diameter, providing valuable additional information by the resulting diagram. The image points on the detection plane are represented by two intensity peaks that must be spatially resolved to discriminate them separately and individually. The peak distance (distance between the functional maxima) and the distortion index (basic diameter of the point cloud in the detection plane) are parameters defined to help understanding when these two peaks are spatially resolved. They help to objectively quantify the individual retinal image in each subject. We found it very useful to evaluate the corneal surface and corneal healing. It is very useful also to explain visual phenomena referred by the patients, and that cannot be explained by older versions of corneal topographers. We don't consider it a substitution of the Eye Sys 2000 Corneal Analysis System (Houston, Texas, USA), but it showed to be a very useful tool.

Subjective symptoms from the pre- and postoperative were noted in the medical report such as haloes, glare, dazzling, corneal and conjunctival dryness, dark-light adaptation and visual satisfaction reported by the patient.

## NONSURGICAL PROCEDURES

### CONTACT LENS MANAGEMENT

Contact lenses are sometimes needed in the postoperative management of refractive surgery. This need arises when it becomes evident to the refractive surgeon that an undesirable result has occurred. The decision of contact lens fitting has to be based on the impossibility of performing new surgeries, or the will of the patient.[5]

## SURGICAL PROCEDURES WITH EXCIMER LASER

We have used different methods for the surgical correction of irregular astigmatism. At this moment we consider three surgical procedures with excimer laser for correction of the irregular astigmatism:

1. **Selective zonal ablation (SELZA)** It is a quantitative method and is useful for improving the irregular astigmatism with defined pattern.[4]

2. **Excimer laser assisted by sodium hyaluronate (ELASHY)** It is a qualitative method. Useful for to improve the irregular astigmatism with undefined pattern.[6]

3. **Topographic linked excimer laser ablation (TOPOLINK)** It is quantitative and qualitative and is useful for improving the irregular astigmatism with defined pattern and the refractive error, with the same procedure.[7]

The surgical procedure was preceded by topical anesthesia of Oxibuprocaine 0.2 percent (Prescaina 0.2%; Laboratorios Llorens, Barcelona, Spain) drops; no patient required sedation. The postoperative treatment consisted of instillation of topical tobramycin 0.3 percent and dexamethasone 0,1 percent drops (Tobradex, Alcon-Cusi, Barcelona, Spain) three times daily for the five days of the follow-up and then discontinued. When the ablation was performed onto the cornea, a bandage contact lens (Actifresh 400, power +0.5, diameter 14.3 mm, radius of curvature 8.8 mm – Hydron Ltd., Hampshire, UK) was used during the first three days of the postoperative and the patient was examined daily. It was removed when complete reepithelialization was observed. Then treatment with topical fluorometholone (FML forte, Alcon-Cusi,

Barcelona, Spain) was used three times daily for the three months of follow-up and then stopped.[8]

Non-preserved artificial tears (Sodium Hyaluronate 0.18%, Vislube®, CHEMEDICA, Ophthalmic line, München, Germany) were used up to three months in every case. Supplementation with oral pain management medications was also used as necessary.

*Statistical analysis* Statistical analysis was performed with the SPSS/Pc+4.0 for Windows (SPSS Inc, Madrid,1996). Measurements typically are reported as the mean $\pm$ 1 standard deviation (using $[n - 1]^{1/2}$ in the denominator of the definition for standard deviation, where n is the number of observations for each measurement) and as the range of all measurements at each follow up visit. Patients' data samples were fitting the normal distribution curves. Statistically significant differences between data sample means were determined by the "t Student's" test; *P* values less than 0.05 were considered significant. Data concerning the standards for reporting the outcome of refractive surgery procedures, as the safety, efficacy and predictability, was analyzed as previously defined.[9]

## SELECTIVE ZONAL ABLATION (SELZA)

In this study we report the results of a prospective clinically controlled study performed on 31 eyes of 26 patients with irregular astigmatism induced by refractive surgery. All cases were treated with SELZA using an excimer laser of broad circular beam (Visx Twenty/Tweenty, 4.02, Visx, Inc. Sunnyvale, California, USA). The surgical planning was applied using the Munnerlyn formula,[10] modified by Buzard,[11] to calculate the depth of the ablation depending on the amount of correction desired and the ablation zone. In this formula the resection depth is equal to the dioptric correction, divided by 3, and multiplied by the ablation zone (mm) squared. We used a correction factor of 1.5 times, to avoid under-correction:

$$\text{Ablation Depth} = \frac{(\text{Dioptric correction}) \times 1.5}{3} \times (\text{ablation zone})^2$$

### Methods

In general, we use ablation zone of 2.5 to 3.0 mm, depending on the steep area of the corneal topography to be modified. The ablation zone was determined by observing the color map. The form of videokeratoscope provides additional information about the irregular zones, and the profile map gave the values for performed ablation. In cases of irregular corneal surface, treatment was performed on the center of irregularity, which was located using the color map of the corneal topography. First we located the center of the cornea, then we located the exact center of irregularity. Here we use the dotted boxes in the map (each dot represents 1 mm$^2$) to detect the exact center of irregularity in relation to the center of the cornea. The amount of ablation is determined using the cross section of the profile map (vertical line corresponding to diopters and horizontal line corresponding to corneal diameter). When the patient had LASIK previously we lift the flap or we do a new LASIK cut and after we perform excimer laser using PTK mode.

The technique is based on subtraction of tissues to eliminate the induced irregular astigmatism and to achieve an uniform corneal surface using excimer laser; we center the effect of laser on zones where the corneal surface is steeper.

### *Discussion*

The selective zonal ablations technique showed satisfactory results on the correction of irregular astigmatism with a defined topographic pattern. Visual acuity improved in the postoperative period, achieving values near to initial BCVA which the patient showed before the initial surgical procedure. The corneal uniformity index evaluating the 3 mm in central diameter, showed improvement in the early postoperative period and stabilising after 3 months, just as the issues of visual acuity ($p < 0.005$). Normally, this refractive procedure requires a stable corneal topography and its adequate interpretation.[12] However, our results have proven that not all irregular astigmatism can be corrected by this method.

## EXCIMER LASER ASSISTED BY SODIUM HYALURONATE (ELASHY)

We report the results of a prospective clinically controlled study performed on 50 eyes of 50 patients with irregular astigmatism.[6] All the patients had been subjected previously to one or more of the following procedures: LASIK, Incisional keratotomy, Photorefractive keratotomy,

Phototherapeutic keratotomy, Laser thermokeratoplasty, and Corneal trauma. Irregular astigmatism was induced thereafter.

Six months after the last corneal procedure, for the aim of stability, the cases were selected for ELASHY.

## Methods

The correction of irregular astigmatism was made with a Plano Scan Technolas 217 C-LASIK Scanning-spot Excimer laser (Bausch and Lomb, Chiron Technolas GmbH, Doranch, Germany) in PTK mode, assisted by viscous masking sodium hyaluronate 0.25 percent solution (LASERVIS® CHEMEDICA, Ophthalmic line, München, Germany). The physical characteristics of sodium hyaluronate confer important rheological properties to the product. The photoablation rate is similar to that of corneal tissue, forming a stable and uniform coating on the surface of the eye, filling depressions on the cornea and effectively masking tissues to be protected against ablation by the laser pulses.[13,14]

In cases where the irregular astigmatism was induced by a flap irregularity or superficial corneal scarring, ELASHY ablations were performed onto the corneal surface. The epithelium was also removed using the excimer laser assisted by viscous masking. When the irregularity was inside the stroma, at the previous stromal bed, the previous flap was lifted up whenever possible or a new cut was done. Then ELASHY was performed at the stroma and after the procedure the flap was repositioned.

We centered the ablation area at the corneal center and fixed it with the eye-tracking device in the center of the pupillary area. After this, one drop of the viscous masking and fluorescein was scattered on the cornea that should be ablated and spread out with the 23-G cannula (Alcon Laboratories, USA) used for the viscous substance instillation. With fluorescein, it was also possible to observe the spot and the effect of laser. Because fluorescent light is emitted during ablation of corneal tissue, cessation of the fluorescence signifies complete removal of the viscous masking solution, i.e. tissue ablation. The laser was prepared for ablation at 15 microns intervals. After each of the intervals, a new drop of the viscous substance was added at the center of the ablation area and again spread out with the same maneuvers with the 23-G cannula. Total treatment was calculated to ablate the prominent areas to the calculated K value at the 4 to 6 mm optical zone or calculated from the tangential map of the Technomed topographer. Assuming a decrease in the ablative effect of the laser due to the use of the viscous agent, we target at a 50% more ablation than the one that corresponds to the real ablation depth necessary for the smoothing procedure.

## Discussion

The results of the study show that the excimer laser plano Scan surgery assisted by sodium hyaluronate 0.25 percent (LASERVIS® CHEMEDICA, Ophthalmic line, München, Germany) (ELASHY) is a useful tool for the treatment of irregular astigmatism, both with and without defined pattern. The clinical indications include irregular astigmatism caused by irregularity in flap or irregularity on stromal base induced by laser *in situ* keratomileusis (LASIK).

Excimer laser application in PTK mode may be undertaken to improve various visual symptoms through improving the corneal surface.[15,17] PTK also can help in cases of irregularities and opacities on corneal surface or anterior stroma, induced by LASIK. In 1994, Gibralter and Trokel applied excimer laser in PTK mode to treat a surgically induced irregular astigmatism in two patients. They used the corneal topographic maps to plan focal treatment areas with good results.[2] The correction of irregular astigmatism should be considered one of these therapeutic indications.

The use of a viscous masking agent should increase the efficiency of the procedure, through protection of the valleys between the irregular corneal peaks, leaving these peaks of pathology exposed to laser treatment. In this study, we used the sodium hyaluronate 0.25 percent (LASERVIS® CHEMEDICA, Ophthalmic line, München, Germany) for this purpose. When the treatment is performed on corneal surface, Bowman's membrane is removed. However, the new epithelium was able to grow and adhere well to the residual stroma. Interestingly, none of our patients developed postoperative haze–normally seen after PRK-, even those subjected to surface treatment. We suggest this effect could be due to the protective properties of the viscoelastic agent, sodium hyaluronate

0.25 percent (LASERVIS® CHEMEDICA, Ophthalmic line, München, Germany), against the oxidative free radical tissue damage.[18]

Many authors have evaluated different masking agents.[13,14] Methylcellulose is the most commonly used agent and is available in different concentrations. Some properties of the methylcellulose, such as to turn white during ablation due to its low boiling point, make this substance not ideal for the purpose of this study.

We found sodium hyaluronate 0.25 percent (LASERVIS® CHEMEDICA, Ophthalmic line, München, Germany) the most suitable for our purpose. It has a photoablation rate similar to that of the corneal tissue. Its stability on the corneal surface forms a uniform coating that fills the depressions on the cornea, protecting them against ablation by the laser pulses.[13] Adding fluorescein to the viscous masking solution is very useful to observe the excimer laser action during corneal ablation at the corneal surface. With experience, it is very easy to distinguish between the ablated areas (in dark) and the marked areas (in green) while the laser radiation is ablating the cornea during the treatment.

The actual corneal ablation is equal to 63 percent of the ablation depth programmed in the software of the excimer laser.[19] If the corneal surface has a masking agent, the initial effect of the laser will be ablating the viscous masking.

The viscous masking solution functions to shield the tissues partially with the faster ablation rate from the laser pulses. Multiple applications of viscous masking solution often are required, and a familiarity with the ablation characteristics will be learned with experience. When the laser ablation is performed on corneal surface, we increase the ablation by 50 mm, necessary for the epithelium ablation.[20]

ELASHY was originally designed for the correction of those irregular astigmatism cases that did not show a pattern and were not available to SELZA correction, yet it proved to be as effective in cases with pattern irregular astigmatism.

Ray-Tracing improved considerably, coinciding with the improvement of the visual subjective symptoms. The superficial corneal surface quality and image distortion were improved, achieving values significantly better than the preoperative values. This demonstrates that a relationship exists between the quality of the corneal surface and the quality of the vision. When the corneal surface is smoothened, the halos, glare and refractive symptoms improve.[21]

## TOPOGRAPHIC LINKED EXCIMER LASER ABLATION (TOPOLINK)

About forty percent of human corneas show some irregularities that cannot be taken into account in a standard basis treatment with excimer laser.[22] For these patients, and for those suffering an irregular astigmatism after trauma or refractive surgery, a custom-tailored, topography-based ablation, which has been adapted to the corneal irregularity, would be the best approach to improve not only their refractive problem but also to improve their quality of vision.

This treatment aims at obtaining the best corrected visual acuity that can be attained by wearing hard contact lenses. It requires an excimer laser with spot scanning technology, in which a small laser spot-by delivering a multitude of single shots fired in diverse positions—is used to create the desired ablation profile. The laser spot is programmable, thus any profile could be created. A videokeratography system that provides an elevation map at high resolution is needed, and specific software is used to create a customized ablation program for the spot scanner laser.

## *Methods*

The aim of this study was to create a regular corneal surface in 41 eyes of 41 patients with irregular astigmatism induced by LASIK: 27 eyes (51.9%) had irregular astigmatism with a defined pattern; 14 eyes (48.1%) had irregular astigmatism without a defined pattern.

All cases were treated with a Plano Scan Technolas 217 C-LASIK Scanning-spot Excimer laser (Bausch and Lomb, Chiron Technolas GmbH, Doranch, Germany) assisted by a C-SCAN Color-Ellipsoid-Topometer (Tech-nomed GmbH, Germany). We performed several corneal topographies from same eye; the software of the auto-mated corneal topographer selected the four exactly equals. These corneal maps, the refractive error, the pachymetry value and desired k-readings calculated for each patient were sent to Technolas by modem. The information was analyzed and a special software program for each patient was created, including it in the Technolas 217 C-LASIK excimer laser by system modem.

The basis for the topography assisted procedure was the preoperative topography.[7,23] This data was transferred into true height data and the treatment for correcting the refractive values in sphere and astigmatism, taking into account the corneal irregularities, was calculated. After that, a postoperative topography was simulated. With this technique, real customized treatment becomes reality, not only treating the refractive error but also improving the patient's visual acuity.

## Discussion

Using the corneal topographic map as a guide, excimer laser ablation can be used to create a more regular surface with improved visual acuity. In a program consisting of a combination of phototherapeutic and photorefractive ablation patterns, the amount of tissue to be removed is calculated on the basis of the diameter and steepness of the irregular areas of the corneal surface. At present, customized ablation based on topography can improve spectacle-corrected visual acuity.

Limitations for this technique exist. With this procedure some irregular astigmatisms cannot be corrected. Some patients could not be selected as candidates for Topolink because any of the following criteria were present:

1. Difference between steep and flat meridians more than 10 D at the 6.0 mm treatment area.
2. Corneal pachymetry was not thick enough (< 400 mm).
3. Diameter of the corneal topography more than 5.0 mm.
4. Corneal topography showing an irregular astigmatism with undefined pattern (irregularly irregular).

This preliminary study showed that topographic-assisted LASIK (Topolink) could be a useful tool to treat irregular astigmatism. This technique is still at an early stage of development. The surgeon depends only on the Placido topographic images, their precision and their reproducibility. Future studies, with more reliable instruments (elevation topography, aberrometer, etc.) will give us the opportunity to deal not only with irregular astigmatism, but also to offer a tailored treatment for all our patients.

## OTHER SURGICAL PROCEDURES

### AUTOMATED ANTERIOR LAMELLAR KERATOPLASTY

This technique was originally designed to treat superficial stromal disorders, but it has also been used for the treatment of difficult cases of irregular astigmatism, with very poor results. The surgeons perform phototherapeutic keratectomy or a microkeratome lamellar resection to 250-400 mm stromal depth, followed by transplantation of a donor lamella of the same dimension on to the recipient bed.[24]

# REFERENCES

1. Azar DT, Strauss I. Principles of applied optics. In Albert DM, Jakobiec FA (Eds): Principles and Practice of Ophthalmology, WB Saunders Co: Philadelphia 1994; 3603-21.

2. Gibralter R, Trokel SL. Correction of irregular astigmatism with the excimer laser. Ophthalmol 1994; 101: 1310-15.

3. Alpins NA. Treatment of irregular astigmatism. J Cataract Refract Surg 1998; 24: 634-46.

4. Alió JL, Artola A, Rodríguez-Mier FA. Selective zonal ablations with excimer laser for correction of irregular astigmatism induced by refractive surgery. Ophthalmol 2000; 107: in press.

5. Zadnik K. Contact lens management of patients who have had unsuccessful refractive surgery. Curr Opin Ophthalmol 1999; 10: 260-63.

6. Alio JL, Belda JI, Shalaby AMM et al. Excimer laser assisted by sodium hyaluronate for correction of irregular astigmatism. Submitted for publication to Ophthalmology 2000.

7. Wiesinger-Jendritza B, Knorz M, Hugger P et al. Laser in situ keratomileusis assisted by corneal topography. J Cataract Surg 1998; 24:166-74.

8. Sher NA, Kreuger RR, Teal P et al. Role of topical corticoids and nonsteroidal anti-inflammatory drugs in the etiology of stromal infiltrates after photorefractive keratectomy. J Refract Corneal Surg 1994; 10: 587-88.

9. Koch DD, Kohnen T, Obstbaum SA et al. Format for reporting refractive surgical data. [letter]. J Cataract Refract Surg 1998; 24: 285-87.

10. Munnerlyn C, Koons S, Marshall J. Photorefractive keratectomy: A technique for laser refractive surgery. J Cataract Refract Surg 1988; 14: 46-52.

11. Buzard K, Fundingsland B. Treament of irregular astigmatism with a broad beam excimer laser. J Refract Surg 1997;13: 624-36.

12. Seitz B, Behrens A, Langenbucher A. Corneal topography. Curr Opin Ophthalmol 1997; 8: 8-24.

13. Kornmehl EW, Steiner RF, Puliafito CA. A comparative study of masking fluids for excimer laser phototherapeutic keratectomy. Arch Ophthalmol 1991;109: 860-63.

14. Kornmehl EW, Steinert RF, Puliafito CA et al. Morphology of an irregular corneal surface following 193 nm ArF excimer laser large area ablation with 0.3% hydroxypropyl methylcellulose 2910 and 0.1% dextran 70.1% carboxy-methylcellulose sodium or 0.9% saline (ARVO abstracts). Invest Ophthalmol Vis Sci 1990;31: 245.

15. Trokel SL, Srinivasan R, Braren B. Excimer laser surgery of the cornea. Am J Ophthalmol 1983;96: 705-10.

16. Kohnen T, Gimbel H, Green F et al. Consultation section: refractive surgical problem. J Cataract Refract Surg 1999; 25: 608-14.

17. Orndahl M, Fagerholm P, Fitzsimmons T et al. Treatment of corneal dystrophies with excimer laser. Acta Ophthalmol 1994; 72: 235-40.

18. Artola A, Alió JL, Bellot JL et al. Protective properties of viscoelastic substances (sodium hyaluronate and 2% hydroxymethyl cellulose) against experimental free radical damage to the corneal endothelium. Cornea 1993; 12: 109-14.

19. Kreuger RR, Trokel SL. Quantification of corneal ablation by ultraviolet light. Arch Ophthalmol 1986; 103:1741-42.

20. Seiler T, Bendee T, Wollensak J. Ablation rate of human corneal epithelium and Bowman's layer with the excimer laser (193nm). J Refract Corneal Surg 1990; 6: 99-102.

21. Klyce SD, Smolek MK: Corneal topography of excimer laser photorefractive keratectomy. J Cataract Refract Surg 1993; 19:122-30.

22. Bogan SJ, Waring GO III, Ibrahim O et al. Classification of normal corneal topography based on computer-assisted videokeratography. Arch Ophthalmol 1990; 108: 945-49.

23. Dausch D, Schröder E, Dausch S. Topography-controlled excimer laser photorefractive keratectomy. J Refract Surg 2000; 16: 13-22.

24. Melles GRJ, Remeijer L, Geerards AJM et al. The future of lamellar keratoplasty. Curr Opin Ophthalmol 1999; 10: 253-59.

# Chapter 6

# *Corneal Topography in Phakonit with a 5 mm Optic Rollable IOL*

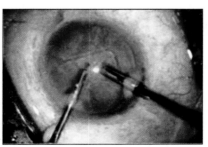

*Amar Agarwal*
*Soosan Jacob*
*Athiya Agarwal*
*Sunita Agarwal*

## INTRODUCTION

Cataract surgery and intraocular lenses (IOL) have evolved greatly since the time of intracapsular cataract extraction and the first IOL implantation by Sir Harold Ridley.[1] The size of the cataract incision has constantly been decreasing from the extremely large ones used for ICCE to the slightly smaller ones used in ECCE to the present day small incisions used in phacoemulsification. Phacoemulsification and foldable IOLs are a major milestone in the history of cataract surgery. Large postoperative against-the-rule astigmatism were an invariable consequence of ICCE and ECCE. This was minimized to a great extent with the 3.2 mm clear corneal incision used for phacoemulsification but nevertheless some amount of residual postoperative astigmatism was a common outcome. The size of the corneal incision was further decreased by Phakonit [2,3,4] a technique introduced for the first time by one of us (Am.A), which separates the infusion from the aspiration ports by utilizing a sleeveless phaco probe and an irrigating chopper. The only limitation to thus realizing the goal of astigmatism neutral cataract surgery was the size of the foldable IOL as the wound nevertheless had to be extended for implantation of the conventional foldable IOLs.

## ROLLABLE IOL

With the availability of the ThinOptX® rollable IOL (Abingdon, VA, USA), that can be inserted through sub-

1.4 mm incision, the full potential of Phakonit could be realized. This lens was created and designed by Wayne Callahan from USA. Subsequently, one of the authors (Am. A) modified the lens by making the optic size 5 mm so that it could go through a smaller incision.

## SURGICAL TECHNIQUE

Five eyes of five patients underwent Phakonit with implantation of an ultrathin 5 mm optic rollable IOL at Dr. Agarwal's Eye Hospital and Eye Research Centre, Chennai. India.

The name PHAKONIT has been given because it shows phacoemulsification (PHAKO) being done with a needle (N) opening via an incision (I) and with the phaco tip (T). A specially designed keratome, an irrigating chopper, a straight blunt rod and a 15° standard phaco tip without an infusion sleeve form the main pre-requisites of the surgery. Viscoelastic is injected with a 26G needle through the presumed site of side port entry. This inflates the chamber and prevents its collapse when the chamber is entered with the keratome. A straight rod is passed through this site to achieve akinesia and a clear corneal temporal valve is made with the keratome **(Figure 6.1A)**. A continuous curvilinear capsulorhexis (CCC) is performed followed by hydrodissection and rotation of the nucleus. After enlarging the side port a 20 Gauge irrigating chopper connected to the infusion line of the phaco

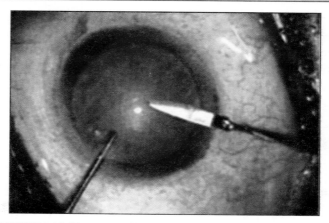

**FIGURE 6.1A:** Clear corneal incision made with a specialized keratome. Note the left hand has a straight rod to stabilize the eye

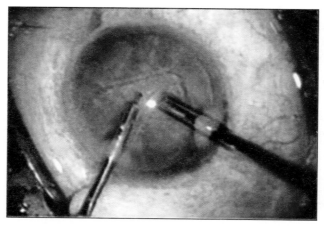

**FIGURE 6.1B:** Agarwal's phakonit irrigating chopper and sleeveless phako probe inside the eye

machine is introduced with foot pedal on position 1. The phaco probe is connected to the aspiration line and the phaco tip without an infusion sleeve is introduced through the main port **(Figure 6.1B)**. Using the phaco tip with moderate ultrasound power, the center of the nucleus is directly embedded starting from the superior edge of rhexis with the phaco probe directed obliquely downwards towards the vitreous. The settings at this stage are 50 percent phaco power, flow rate 24 ml/min and 110 mm Hg vacuum. When nearly half of the center of nucleus is embedded, the foot pedal is moved to position 2 as it helps to hold the nucleus due to vacuum rise. To avoid undue pressure on the posterior capsule the nucleus is lifted slightly and with the irrigating chopper in the left hand the nucleus chopped. This is done with a straight downward motion from the inner edge of the rhexis to the center of the nucleus and then to the left in the form of an inverted L shape. Once the crack is created, the nucleus is split till the center. The nucleus is then rotated 180° and cracked again so that the nucleus is completely split into two halves. With the previously described technique, 3 pie-shaped quadrants are created in each half of the nucleus. With a short burst of energy at pulse mode, each pie-shaped fragment is lifted and brought at the level of iris where it is further emulsified and aspirated sequentially in pulse mode. Thus the whole nucleus is removed. Cortical wash-up is then done with the bimanual irrigation aspiration technique.

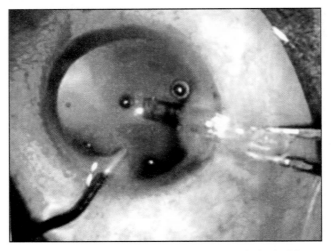

***FIGURE 6.1C:*** The rollable IOL inserted through the incision

The lens is taken out from the bottle and placed in a bowl of BSS solution of approximately body temperature to make the lens pliable. It is then rolled with the gloved hand holding it between the index finger and the thumb. The lens is then inserted through the incision carefully **(Figure 6.1C)**. The tear drop on the haptic should be pointing in a clockwise direction so that the smooth optic lenticular surface faces posteriorly. The natural warmth of the eye causes the lens to open gradually. Viscoelastic is then removed with the bimanual irrigation aspiration probes **(Figure 6.1D)**. **Figure 6.1** shows different steps of the surgery.

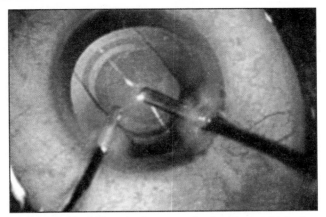

***FIGURE 6.1D:*** Vviscoelastic removed using bimanual irrigation aspiration probes

## TOPOGRAPHIC ANALYSIS AND ASTIGMATISM

The preoperative best-corrected visual acuity (BCVA) ranged from 20/60 to 20/200. The mean preoperative. astigmatism as detected by topographic analysis was 0.98 D ± 0.62 D ( range 0.5 to 1.8 D).

The postoperative course was uneventful in all cases. The IOL was well-centered in the capsular bag. There were no corneal burns in any of the cases.

Four eyes had a best-corrected visual acuity of 20/30 or better. One eye that had dry ARMD showed an improvement in BCVA from 20/200 to 20/60. **Figure 6.2** shows a comparison of the pre and postoperative BCVA. The mean astigmatism on postoperative day 1 on topographic analysis was 1.1 ± 0.61 D (range 0.6 to 1.9 D) as

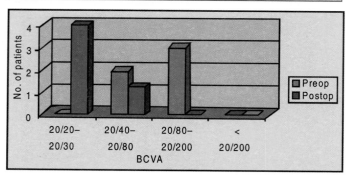

**FIGURE 6.2:** Comparison of pre and postoperative BCAV

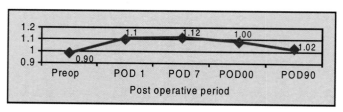

**FIGURE 6.3:** Mean astigmatism over-time

compared to 0.98 D ± 0.62 D ( range 0.5 to 1.8 D) preoperatively. The mean astigmatism was 1.02 ± 0.64 D ( range 0.3 to 1.7 D) by 3 months post operatively. **Figures 6.3 and 6.4** show mean astigmatism over time. **Figures 6.5A and 6.5B** show a comparison of the astigmatism over the pre and post surgical period.

## DISCUSSION

Cataract surgery has witnessed great advancements in surgical technique, foldable IOLs and phaco technology.

| Time | Eyes | Mean | Std. Dev. | Minimum | Maximum |
|------|------|------|-----------|---------|---------|
| Preop | 5 | 0.98 | 0.62 | 0.5 | 1.8 |
| POD 1 | 5 | 1.1 | 0.61 | 0.6 | 1.9 |
| POD 7 | 5 | 1.12 | 0.58 | 0.5 | 1.7 |
| POD 30 | 5 | 1.08 | 0.62 | 0.5 | 1.8 |
| POD 90 | 5 | 1.02 | 0.64 | 0.3 | 1.7 |

*FIGURE 6.4:* Table showing pre and postoperative mean astigmatism

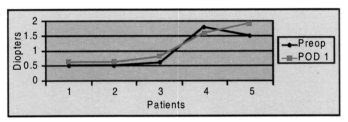

*FIGURE 6.5A:* Comparison of pre and post operative day 1 cylinder

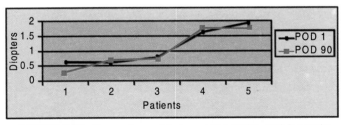

*FIGURE 6.5B:* Comparison of 1 day postoperative and 3 months postoperative astigmatism

This has made possible easier and safer cataract extraction utilizing smaller incision. With the advent of the latest IOL technology which enables implantation through ultrasmall incisions, it is clear that this will soon replace routine phacoemulsification through the standard 3.2 mm incisions. The ThinOptX® IOL design is based on the Fresnel principle. This was designed by Wayne Callahan (USA). Flexibility and good memory are important characteristics of the lens. It is manufactured from hydrophilic acrylic materials and is available in a range from −25 to +30 with the lens thickness ranging from 30 $\mu$m up to 350 $\mu$m. One of the authors (Am.A) has modified the lens further by reducing the optic size to 5 mm to go through a smaller incision. The lens is now undergoing clinical-trials in Europe and the USA.

In this study, no intraoperative complications were encountered during CCC, phacoemulsification, cortical aspiration or IOL lens insertion in any of the cases. The mean phacoemulsification time was 0.66 minutes. Previous series by the same authors showed more than 300 eyes where cataract surgery was successfully performed using the sub-1 mm incision.[3] Our experience and that of several other surgeons suggests that with existing phacoemulsification technology, it is possible to perform phacoemulsification through ultra-small incisions without significant complications[2-6]. In a recent study from Japan, Tsuneoka and associates[6] used a sleeveless phaco tip to perform bimanual phacoemulsification in 637 cataractous eyes. All cataracts were safely removed by these authors through an incision of 1.4 mm or smaller that was widened for IOL insertion, without a case of thermal burn and with few intraoperative complications. Furthermore, ongoing research for the development of laser probes[7,8] cold phaco, and microphaco confirms the interest of leading ophthalmologists and manufacturers in the direction of ultra-small incisional cataract surgery (Fine IN, Olson RJ, Osher RH, Steinert RF. Cataract technology makes strides. Ophthalmology Times, December 1, 2001, pp 12-15).

The postoperative course was uneventful in all the cases. The IOL was well centered in the capsular bag. There were no significant corneal burns in any of the cases. Final visual outcome was satisfactory with 4 of the eyes having a BCVA of 20/30 or better. One eye that had dry ARMD showed an improvement in BCVA from 20/200 to 20/60. Thus the lens was found to have satisfactory optical performance within the eye. In our study, the mean astigmatism on topographical analysis was $0.98 \pm 0.62$ D (range 0.5 to 1.8 D) preoperatively, $1.1 \pm 0.61$ D (range 0.6 to 1.9 D) on postoperative day 1 and $1.02 \pm 0.64$ D (range 0.3 to 1.7 D) by 3 months post operatively. **Figures 6.5A and 6.5B** showing a comparison of the pre and postoperative astigmatism indicate clearly that Phakonit with an ultrathin 5 mm rollable IOL is virtually astigmatically neutral. **Figures 6.6A and 6.6B** depicting the topography comparison in different surgical periods show clearly the virtual astigmatic neutrality of the procedure and stability throughout the postoperative course.

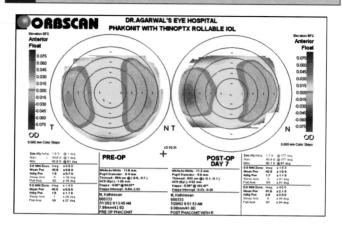

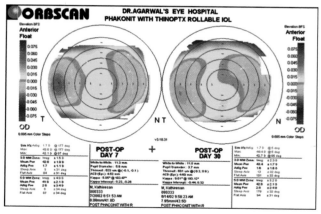

**FIGURE 6.6:** Topographical comparison during different surgical periods

There is an active ongoing attempt to develop newer IOLs that can go through smaller and smaller incisions. Phakonit ThinOptX® modified ultrathin rollable IOL is the first prototype IOL which can go through sub-1.4 mm incisions. Research is also in progress to manufacture this IOL using hydrophobic acrylic biomaterials combined with square-edged optics to minimize posterior capsule opacification.

## CONCLUSION

Phakonit with an ultrathin 5 mm optic rollable IOL implantation is a safe and effective technique of cataract extraction, the greatest advantage of this technique being virtual astigmatic neutrality.

## REFERENCES

1. Apple DJ, Auffarth GU, Peng Q, Visessook N. Foldable Intraocular Lenses. Evolution, Clinicopathologic Correlations, Complications. Thorofare, NJ, Slack , Inc., 2000.
2. Agarwal A, Agarwal A, Agarwal S, et al. Phakonit: Phacoemulsification through a 0.9 mm corneal incision. J Cataract Refract Surg 2001; 27:1548-52.
3. Agarwal A, Agarwal A, Agarwal A, et al. Phakonit: Lens removal through a 0.9 mm incision. (Letter). J Cataract Refract Surg 2001; 27:1531-32.
4. Agarwal A, Agarwal S, Agarwal A. Phakonit and laser phaconit: Lens removal through a 0.9 mm incision. In: Agarwal S, Agarwal A, Sachdev MS, Fine IH, Agarwal A, editors, Phacoemulsification, laser cataract surgery and foldable IOLs. New Delhi, India, Jaypee, 2000; 204-16.
5. Tsuneoka H, Shiba T, Takahashi Y. Feasibility of ultrasound cataract surgery with a 1.4 mm incision. J Cataract Refract Surg 2001; 27:934-40.
6. Tsuneoka H, Shiba T, Takahashi Y. Ultrasonic phacoemulsification using a 1.4 mm incision: Clinical results. J Cataract Refract Surg 2002;28:81-86.

7. Kanellpoupolos AJ. A prospective clinical evaluation of 100 consecutive laser cataract procedures using the Dodick photolysis neodymium: Yittrium-aluminum-garnet system. Ophthalmology 2001;108:1-6.

8. Dodick JM. Laser phacolysis of the human cataractous lens. Dev Ophthalmol 1991; 22:58-64.

# Chapter 7

# *Topographic and Aberrometer-guided Laser*

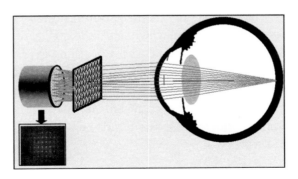

*Amar Agarwal*
*Sunita Agarwal*
*Athiya Agarwal*

## INTRODUCTION

Since as early as middle of 19th century it has been known that the optical quality of human eye suffers from ocular errors (aberrations) besides the commonly known image errors such as myopia, hyperopia and astigmatism.[1] In early 1970's Fyodorov introduced the anterior radial incisions to flatten the central cornea to correct myopia.[2] Astigmatic keratotomy,[3] Keratomileusis and Keratophakia, Epikeratophakia[4] and currently Excimer Laser[5] have been used to manage the various refractive errors. These refractive procedures correct lower order aberrations such as spherical and cylindrical refractive errors however higher order aberrations persist, which affect the quality of vision but may not significantly affect the Snellen visual acuity. Refractive corrective procedures are known to induce aberrations.[6] It is the subtle deviations from the ideal optical system, which can be corrected by wavefront and topography guided (customized ablation) LASIK procedures.[7]

## ABERRATIONS

Optical aberration customization can be corneal topography guided which measures the ocular aberrations detected by corneal topography and treats the irregularities as an integrated part of the laser treatment plan. The second method of optical aberration customization measures the wavefront errors of the entire eye and treats based on these measurements.[7] Wavefront analysis can be done either using Howland's aberroscope[8] or a Hartmann Shack wavefront sensor.[9] These techniques measure all the *eye*'s aberrations including second-order (sphere and cylindrical), third-order (coma–like), fourth-order (spherical), and higher order wavefront aberrations. Based on this information an ideal ablation plan can be formulated which treats lower order as well as higher order aberrations.

## ZYOPTIX LASER

Zyoptix™ (Bausch and Lomb) is a system for Personalized Vision Solutions, which incorporates Zywave ™ Hartmann Shack aberrometer coupled with Orbscan ™ II z multi-dimensional device, which generates the individual ablation profiles to be used with the Technolas® 217 Excimer Laser System. Thus this system utilizes combination of wavefront analysis and corneal topography for optical aberration customization.

## ORBSCAN

The Orbscan (BAUSCH & LOMB) corneal topography system uses a scanning optical slit-scan that is fundamentally different than the corneal topography that analyses the reflected images from the anterior corneal surface. The high-resolution video camera captures 40 light-slits at 45 degrees angle projected through the cornea similarly as seen during slit lamp examination. The slits are projected on to the anterior segment of the eye: the anterior cornea, the posterior cornea, the anterior iris and anterior lens. The data collected from these four surfaces are used to create a topographic map. This technique provides more information about anterior segment of the eye, such as anterior and posterior corneal curvature and corneal thickness.[10] It improves the diagnostic accuracy and it has passive eye-tracker from frame to frame, 43 frames are taken to ensure accuracy. It is easy to interpret and has good repeatability. Three different maps are taken, and the one featuring the least eye movements is used. The maximum movements considered acceptable are $200\mu$.

## ABERROMETER

Zywave™ is based on Hartmann-Shack aberrometry **(Figure 7.1)** in which a laser diode (780 nm) generates a laser beam that is focused on the retina of the patient's eye **(Figure 7.2)**. An adjustable collimation system compensates for the spherical portion of the refractive error of the eye. Laser diode is turned on for approximately 100 milliseconds. The light reflected from the focal point on the retina (source of wavefront) is directed through an array of small lenses (lenslet) generating a grid like pattern (array) of focal points **(Figure 7.3)**. The position of the focal points are detected by Zywave™ .Due to deviation of the points from their ideal position, the wavefront can be reconstructed. Wavefront display shows (a) higher order aberrations (b) predicted phoropter refraction (PPR) calculated for a back vertex correction of 15 mm, (c) simulated point spread function (PSF).

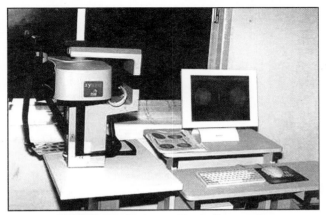

*FIGURE 7.1:* Hartmann-Shack Aberrometer

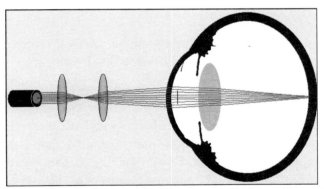

*FIGURE 7.2:* Zywave projects low-intensity He, Ne infrared light into the eye and uses the diffuse reflection from the retina

Zywave™ examinations are done with (a) single examination with undilated pupil (b) five examinations with dilated pupil (mydriasis) non-cycloplegic, using 5 percent Phenylephrine drops. One of these five measure-

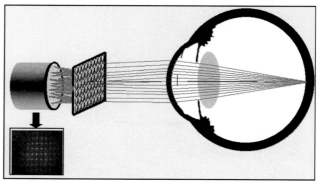

**FIGURE 7.3:** Schematic illustration of the Bausch and Lomb Zywave aberrometer. A low-intensity He, Ne infrared light is shone into the eye; the reflected light is focused by a number of small lenses (lenslet-array), and pictured by a CCD-camera. The captured image is shown on the bottom left

ments, which matched best with the manifest refraction of the undilated pupil, is chosen for the treatment.

## ZYLINK

Information gathered from Orbscan and Zywave are then translated into treatment plan using Zylink™ software and copied to a floppy disc. The floppy disc is then inserted into the Technolas 217 system **(Figure 7.4)**, fluence test carried out and a Zyopitx treatment card was inserted. A standard LASIK procedure is then performed with a superiorly hinged flap. A Hansatome™ microkeratome is used to create a flap. Flap thickness varied from 160 $\mu$m to 200 $\mu$m. A residual stromal bed of 250 $\mu$m or more is left in all eyes. Optical zone varied from 6 mm to 7 mm

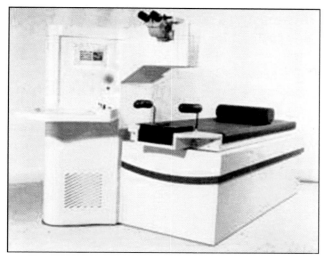

***FIGURE 7.4:*** Technolas 217 z excimer laser system.

depending upon the pupil size and ablation required. Eye tracker is kept on during laser ablation. Postoperatively all patients are followed up for at least 6 months.

## RESULTS

We did a study comprising 150 eyes with myopia and compound myopic astigmatism. Pre-operatively, the patients underwent corneal topography with Orbscan IIz™ and wavefront analysis with Zywave ™ in addition to the routine pre-LASIK work up. The results were assimilated using Zylink ™ and a customized treatment plan was formulated. LASIK was then performed with Technolas®

217 system. All the patients were followed up for at least six months.

Mean pre-operative BCVA (in decimal) was 0.83 ± 0.18 (Range 0.33- 1.00). Mean post-operative (6 months) BCVA was 1.00 ± 0.23 (Range 0.33-1.50). Difference was statistically significant (p=0.0003). Out of 150 eyes that underwent customized ablation, 3 eyes (2%) lost two or more lines of best spectacle corrected visual acuity (BSCVA).

Safety Index = Mean post-operative BSCVA / Mean pre-operative BSCVA = 1.20 **(Figure 7.5)**. Mean pre-operative UCVA was 0.06 ± 0.02 (Range 0.01-0.50). Mean post-operative UCVA was 0.88 ± 0.36 (Range 0.08 – 1.50). Difference was statistically significant (p =0.0001).

Efficacy index = Mean post-operative UCVA / Mean pre-operative UCVA = 14.66 **(Figure 7.6)**. Pre-operatively, none of the eyes had UCVA of 6\6 or more and one eye (0.66%) had UCVA of 6/12 or more. At 6 months post-operatively, 105 eyes (69.93%) had UCVA of 6\6 or more and 126 eyes (83.91%) had UCVA of 6/12 or more.

Mean pre-operative spherical equivalent was -5.25 D ± 1.68 D (Range –0.87 D to –15 D). Mean post-operative spherical equivalent (6 months) was –0.36 D ± 0.931 D (Range –4.25 D to +1.25). Difference between the two was statistically significant (p<0.05) **(Figure 7.7)**. 132 eyes (87.91%) were within ±1.00 D of emmetropia while 120 eyes (79.92%) were within ± 0.05 D of emmetropia. 1 eye (0.66%) was overcorrected by > 0.5 D and 1 eye

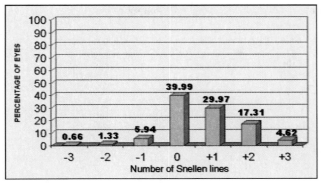

***FIGURE 7.5:*** Shows changes in BSCVA 6 months post-operatively
(Safety)

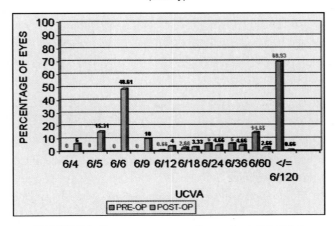

***FIGURE 7.6:*** Compares preoperative and postoperative
UCVA (Efficacy)

(0.66%) was overcorrected by >1D. The mean pupil
diameter was 5.1mm ± 0.62mm. Preoperatively, 95 eyes
(63.27%) had third order aberrations.42 eyes (28%) had

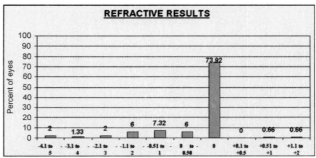

**FIGURE 7.7:** Shows the refractive results post-operatively after 6 months

second order aberration alone, while 13 eyes (8.65%) had fourth and fifth order aberrations. Post-operatively, 60 eyes (40%) had third order aberration. 75 eyes (50%) had second order alone while 15 eyes (10%) had higher order aberrations.

## DISCUSSION

Hartmann-Shack wavefront sensor was first used by Liang and colleagues to detect ocular aberrations.[11] They applied an adaptive optics deformable mirror to correct the lower and higher order aberrations of the eye. They reported a 6 times increase in contrast sensitivity to high spatial frequency when the pupil was large. This study demonstrated that correction of higher order aberrations could lead to supernormal vision in normal eyes.

In our series, using Zyoptix and Technolas 217 system, which is wavefront and corneal topography guided, we yielded results that are comparable to standard LASIK procedure.[12] In a series of 347 eyes, McDonald et al [12] reported a post-operative refraction of $-0.29 \pm 0.45$ D ($-0.36 \pm 0.93$ D in our series) with standard LASIK. 57% of the eyes in their series had post-operative UCVA of $=6/6$. In our study, 70% of the eyes had UCVA of $=6/6$, six months post-operatively.

Higher order aberrations were reduced postoperatively in our study. Third-order aberration (coma) was most common in our series, followed by second-order (defocus and astigmatism) and fourth-order (spherical aberration). Post-operatively, after 6 months, there was considerable decrease in third-order and fourth-order aberrations. While most of the eyes had only defocus and astigmatism (i.e. second -order aberration). A slight increase in fourth-order aberration (spherical) was noted. Spherical aberration is known to increase after LASIK.[13-15] Roberts has reported that cornea changes its shape in response to ablation and this change, along with wound healing effects have to be taken into account before customized correction can nullify higher-order aberrations. Roberts and coworkers suggest that increase in spherical aberrations following LASIK may be caused by a biomechanically induced steepening and thickening that may occur in mid periphery of the cornea.[13] MacRae and coworkers have reported that simply creating a LASIK flap increases higher-order aberrations in unpredictable manner.[14] They suggest that improved results can be obtained using a surface ablation such as PRK or LASEK, or by doing a two-stage LASIK, with the second stage adjusting for the aberration created by the flap and initial ablation.

Scotopic visual complaints have been the bugbear of LASIK procedures, ranging from mild annoyance to server optical disability.[16,17] Night time starbursts, reduced contrast sensitivity and haloes are the most common complaints. [16,17] Spherical aberration that is induced during LASIK may account for this scotopic complaints.[14] Pupil diameter is another factor that is important. When pupil diameter is large, as in young patients, dim light vision is improved after customized correction. [18,19] In our series, 11 percent of the patients complained of haloes around light at night and difficult night driving. In dim light, the mean pupil diameter in these patients was 4.2mm while it was 5.9mm in other patients. Smaller pupil diameter and induced higher-order aberration may account for these scotopic visual complaints.

Twenty-five percent of the patients in our series reported improvement in bright light vision, while 40 percent showed improvement in dim light vision. A similar improvement was noted by Cox and co-workers (presentation by Cox IG at Zyoptix Alliance Meeting, 2002 reported in *Ocular Surgery News*, July 2002 volume 13, number 7). In our series, treatment optical zone ranged from 6mm to 7mm. Treatment with larger optical zones and transition zones as compared to conventional LASIK may be possible since entire corneal topography and not just the central cornea overlying pupil along with wavefront ablation in dilated pupil are considered during treatment. This may induce lesser spherical aberration post-LASIK and account for improved scotopic vision.

Though we did not measure contrast sensitivity and glare acuity post-operatively, our results suggest improved quality of vision and fewer glare problems with Zyoptix treatment. A more temporal appraisal of the procedure has to be carried out with comparison to standard LASIK. Short-term results suggest wavefront and topography guided LASIK may be a safe and effective procedure which improves the visual performance.

## CONCLUSION

Wavefront and topography guided LASIK procedure leads to better visual performance by decreasing higher order aberration. Scotopic visual complaints may be reduced with this method.

## REFERENCES

1. Helmholtz H. Handbuch der physiologischen optik. Leipzig: Leopold Voss. 1867;137-47.
2. Fyodorov S N, Durnev VV. Operation of dosaged dissection of corneal circular ligament.
3. Binder PS, Waring GO III: Keratotomy for astigmatism. In Waring GO III (Ed.): Refractive keratotomy for myopia and astigmatism. Mosby Year Book 1992; 1085–1198. In cases of myopia of mild degree. Ann Ophthalmol II: 1979; 1885–90.
4. Kaufmann HE: Correction of aphakia Am J Ophthalmol 1980; 89.
5. McGhee CNJ, Taylor HR, Garty DS et al. Excimer Lasers in Ophthalmology: Principles and Practice Martin Duntz: London, 1997.
6. MacRae S, Porter J, Cox IG et al. Higher-order aberrations after conventional LASIK. ISRS: Dallas, Texas, 2000.
7. MacRae SM: Supernormal vision, hypervision, and customized corneal ablation. Guest Editorial J Cat Refract Surg 2000; 26(2).

8. Howland HC, Howland B. A subjective method for the measurement of monochromatic aberrations of the eye. J Opt Soc Am 1977; 67:1508-1518

9. Liang J, Williams DR, Miller DT. Supernormal vision and high-resolution retinal imaging through adaptive optics. J Opt Soc Am 1997: 2884-92.

10. Fedor P, Kaufman S. Corneal topography and imaging. Medicine Journal, 2001; 2(6).

11. Liang J, Williams D. Aberrations and retinal image quality of the normal human eye. J Opt Soc AM A 1997;14:2884-2892.

12. McDonald MB, Carr JD, Frantz JM, et al. Laser in situ keratomilieusis for myopia up to −11 diopters with up to −5 diopters of astigmatism with summit autonomous LADAR Vision excimer laser system. Ophthalmology 2001;108:309-316.

13. Roberts C. The cornea is not a piece of plastic. J Refract Surg 2000;16:407-413.

14. MacRae SM, Roberts C, Porter J, et al. The biomechanics of a LASIK flap. ISRS Mid-Summer Meeting: Orlando, Florida, 2001.

15. Applegate RA, Howland HC, Klyce SD. Corneal aberration and refractive surgery. In: MacRae S (Eds). Customized Corneal Ablation. Thorofare NJ: Slack, Inc., 2001.

16. Holladay JT, Dudeja DR, Chang J. Functional vision and corneal changes after laser in situ keratomileusis determined by contrast sensitivity, glare testing, and corneal topography. J Cataract Refract Surg 1999; 25: 663-69.

17. Perez-Santonja JJ, Sakla HF, Alio JL. Contrast sensitivity after laser in situ keratomileusis. J Cataract Refract Surg 1998; 24: 183-9.

18. Applegate R, Howland H, Sharp R, et al. Corneal aberrations and visual performance after refractive keratectomy. J Refract Surg 1998; 14: 397-407.

19. Oshika T, Klyce S, Applegate R, et al. Comparison of corneal wavefront aberrations after photorefractive keratectomy and laser in situ keratomileusis. Am J Ophthal 1999; 127:1-7.

# Chapter 8

# *Topography-assisted LASIK*

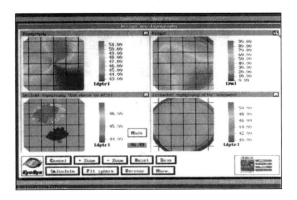

*Michael C Knorz*
*Maria C Arbelaez*

## INTRODUCTION

The invention of excimer lasers led to a tremendous improvement in the predictability of refractive surgical procedures. By moving the ablation inside the cornea, the introduction of laser-in-situ keratomileusis (LASIK) virtually eliminated scarring and regression, making it possible to treat high myopia as well as hyperopia. By adding LASIK to their spectrum, refractive surgeons were able to treat almost any refractive error.

Besides myopia, hyperopia, and astigmatism, we all know the rare cases with grossly irregular patterns following, e.g. penetrating corneal grafts, penetrating injuries, or peripheral corneal scars that cause irregularity. All these eyes could be treated rather unsuccessfully to date. In these eyes, we wished we had a software to custom-tailor the ablation and that is exactly what topography-assisted LASIK, (TA-LASIK) is about.

A custom-tailored ablation is also extremely useful and ultimately even more important in slight corneal asymmetries. Today, we use standardized and symmetrical ablation pattern, which is similar to buying a suit "off-the-rack". The individual corneas of our patients, however, show a lot of asymmetry. As many as 40 percent of eyes show some degree of asymmetry, and all these eyes would be far better off with a customised laser ablation. TA-LASIK is the ideal tool to create a perfect cornea as it allows us to reshape the cornea in any pattern we may decide. All that is required is corneal topography (Technomed C-Scan or EyeSys), the proprietary software, a Hansatome microkeratome (Bausch and Lomb Surgical), and a Keracor 117C or 217 excimer laser from Bausch and Lomb Surgical.

## HOW DOES TA-LASIK WORK?

**As in all refractive procedures, the first requirement to be met is stability of the cornea. It does not make sense to operate as long as the shape of the cornea is still changing.** There should be a time interval of at least one year following penetrating grafts or large penetrating injuries. In small scars, of course, the interval could be shorter. Whenever uncertain, the surgeon should wait for three months and reexamine the patient. Now, as soon as the cornea is stable, a corneal topography is taken in the routine fashion. This topographic map should be of as high a quality as possible because it is used as the basis of the ablation. This means that the lids are wide open, that the tear film is regular, that there are no "dark spots" on the map, that the picture is well centered and well focused, and that the entrance pupil is visible on the map. All these requirements are easy to meet for experienced observers in normal corneas, but sometimes quite difficult in abnormal ones, which are the corneas we will treat with TA-LASIK. If it is not possible to obtain a good picture, the examination should be repeated at a later date. It is also a good idea to perform topography prior to any other examinations. In addition, we learned from mistakes in the beginning and now require a set of three topographic maps taken at the same day to calculate the ablation.

Assuming perfect maps were obtained, the respective data files are exported onto a disk which is either physically or electronically transferred to Bausch and Lomb Surgical Technolas, Munich, Germany. This procedure is state-of-the-art even today. Later on, the required software will definitely be available either on the laser or on the topography unit. The respective software then converts measurements of radii of curvature to true height values. Based on the height, the ablation is calculated by a proprietary algorithm. All we have to do is to tell the software which K-value it should target. This is another tricky issue in very irregular corneas, but only the correct K-value will create an emmetropic eye and therefore an extremely happy patient. Should the K-value not be accurate, however, this will result in some spherical deviations from emmetropia which is still much better than an irregular cornea. To establish the actual K-value of a specific cornea, we used topographic maps (normalized scale) and subjectively estimated the average refractive power of the part of the cornea overlying the entrance pupil. In irregular corneas, this requires some guessing.

In addition to the K-value, we must provide the diameter of the desired ablation zone and, of course, pachymetry of the central cornea. Pachymetry is especially important in repair procedures following previous refractive surgery, e.g. PRK (photorefractive keratectomy) or LASIK. The cornea is thinner after PRK or LASIK, which leaves less space for further ablations. Therefore, it is very important to measure corneal thickness in these cases.

After all parameters are set, the computer will calculate a treatment based on the corneal topography of the individual eye.

## CASE REPORTS

### PATIENT CW: IRREGULAR ASTIGMATISM AFTER PENETRATING INJURY

This 6-year-old patient had suffered a penetrating injury in her left eye. A light bulb exploded, and glass fragments penetrated her eye, causing corneal lacerations extending from 10 to 12 O'clock peripherally. One year after the initial repair, scar formation caused significant irregular astigmatism. Uncorrected visual acuity (UCVA) was 20/200. With a correction of +0.5 sphere –5.0 cyl axis 170°, an acuity of 20/100 was achieved. Contact lenses were tried but not tolerated by the patient. Corneal topography showed marked irregular astigmatism. Therefore, the authors discussed treatment options with the parents of this child. As contact lenses were not tolerated, surgery seemed to be the only option to prevent amblyopia. We considered T-cuts, corneal grafts and TA-LASIK. LASIK was selected as the least invasive and most predictable option. Surgery was performed under general anesthesia. **Figure 8.1** shows the topographic work place on which the ablation is planned. The preoperative topographic map (scale in diopters) is on the upper left, and the ablation profile suggested by the TA-LASIK software (scale in mm) on the upper right. On the lower left, the surgeon can

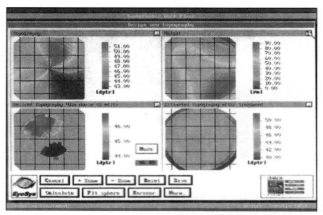

***FIGURE 8.1:*** Topographic workplace used to design the ablation of patient CW. The preoperative topographic map (scale in diopters) is on the upper left, and the ablation profile suggested by the TA-LASIK software (scale in µm) on the upper right. On the lower left, the surgeon can add individual fudge factors, and the expected result is displayed on the lower right hand side

add individual fudge factors, and the expected result is displayed on the lower right hand side. Comparing maps, we can see that the flat area at the lower right (blue colors) of the preoperative topography map is steepened by the ablation (red color at the lower right of the ablation map). Superposing the two maps in the upper row, the resulting map, which is displayed at the lower right, should be a perfect sphere, at least theoretically.

**Figure 8.2** shows the results of the calculated ablation we just described. The preoperative topographic map and the topographic map one day after surgery are shown in **Figure 8.2**. The color scale is the same in both maps, which can therefore directly be compared. As clearly

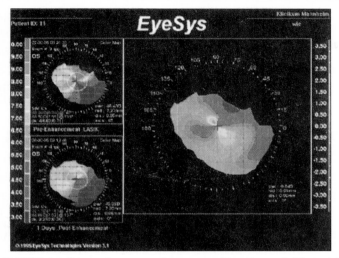

**FIGURE 8.2:** Pre- and postoperative topographic maps and differential map of patient CW (penetrating injury with irregular astigmatism)

visible, the steep area on the upper left is considerably flatter, and visual acuity without correction improved to 20/60 on day one. **Figure 8.2** also shows the differential map. The change map, which visualizes the ablation that was performed, closely resembles the planned ablation (see **Figure 8.1**, upper right, for comparison). One year after surgery, visual acuity without correction was 20/80, and with correction of –2 cyl axis 140° acuity was 20/60. To prevent amblyopia, the right eye was occluded 4 hours a day. Corneal topography at one year shows considerable regression of effect. The cornea was still more regular than preoperatively, but most of the effect had regressed. We considered a retreatment and calculated an ablation of

50 m. Preoperatively, corneal thickness was 587 m. Flap thickness was 160 m, and ablation depth during the first TA-LASIK procedure was 86 m. Central corneal thickness after the first procedure was 430 m. We therefore decided against a retreatment to avoid possible late keratectasia due to corneal thinning.

## PATIENT AT: DECENTERED ABLATION AFTER PRK

Mr AT is a 40-year-old patient who had PRK in his right eye in July 1994 (Meditec MEL 60 excimer laser). His preoperative refraction was −8 D in his right eye. After PRK, he complained about halos and double vision, most pronounced in dim light and at night, and had refused PRK in his second eye because of these problems. He was referred to us for possible retreatment. Corneal topography revealed a small ablation zone which was also decentered superotemporally (**Figure 8.3**, upper left). The average refractive power of the cornea overlaying the entrance pupil was estimated to be 41 D. UCVA was 20/30, spectacle-corrected visual acuity (SCVA) was 20/20 (−1.0 sphere −1.5 cyl axis 160°). Central corneal thickness was 469 m. We decided to perform TA-LASIK. Considering a corneal refraction of, on average, 41 D and a manifest spherical equivalent (SE) of −1.75 D, we aimed for a target K-value (corneal refraction) of 39 D. Optical zone size was 6 mm, ablation depth 95 m. As a flap thickness of 160 m was used, this left a stromal bed of roughly 200 m which we consider to be the minimum in order to avoid possible late ectasia. Corneal topography

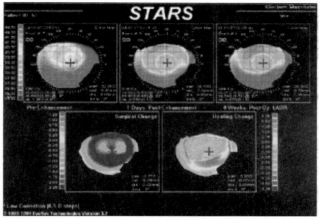

**FIGURE 8.3:** STARS display of patient AT (decentered ablation after PRK). The preoperative map is shown on the upper left, the map on day 1 in the center, and the map at 1 month on the upper right. The differential map on the lower left (surgical change) shows that the ablation zone was enlarged and the central astigmatism was removed. The map on the lower right (healing change) shows some regression of effect, indicated by the steepening (red colors) around the edge of the ablation zone

at day 1 shows a much larger ablation zone (**Figure 8.3**, center). Visual acuity was 20/20 without correction on day one, and the halos had disappeared. Visual acuity and refraction remained stable throughout the postoperative follow-up which is now 6 months. Corneal topography is shown in **Figure 8.3**. The STARS display allows for evaluation of both the surgical change and the healing change, or regression. The differential map on the lower left (surgical change) shows that the ablation zone was enlarged and the central astigmatism was removed. The map on the lower right shows some regression of effect, indicated by the steepening (red colors) around the edge of the ablation zone.

## PATIENT DK: IRREGULAR ASTIGMATISM AFTER PKP AND RK

The patient, a judge at a local court, had had a penetrating corneal graft because of recurrent stromal herpetic keratitis in 1992. He was first referred in 1993. Manifest refraction was +0.25 sphere –6 cyl axis 135°. Corneal astigmatism was –8 D axis 135° and slightly asymmetric. Initially, astigmatic keratotomy was performed in 1994. After AK, manifest refraction was –2.5 sphere –4 cyl axis 165°. UCVA was 20/400 and best-corrected visual acuity (BCVA) was 20/60. Corneal topography showed marked irregularity and axis shift (**Figure 8.4**, upper left). We therefore decided to perform TA-LASIK. Average refractive power of the cornea overlaying the entrance pupil was estimated to be 45 D. Spherical equivalent of manifest refraction was –4.5 D. We therefore selected a target K-value of 40.5 D. A 5.4-mm optical zone was used, and ablation depth was 150 m. Corneal thickness was 610m centrally, and both the internal and external margins of the graft were well aligned with the host cornea. It is very important to check alignment prior to the lamellar cut. In poor alignment or localized ectasia at the edge, corneal thickness might be reduced, and the keratome cut may cause further weakening of the cornea, inducing more ectasia, or even

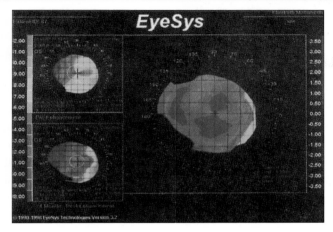

**FIGURE 8.4:** Pre- and postoperative topographic maps and differential map of patient DK (irregular astigmatism after PKP and RK)

a penetration of the anterior chamber. In this patient, alignment was perfect, and the LASIK procedure performed in July 1997 was uneventful. A $160\mu$ flap was used. One day after TA-LASIK, UCVA had improved to 20/30, and BCVA was 20/25 (correction: +0.75 sphere). After 4 months, UCVA was 20/30 and BCVA 20/25, but manifest refraction had changed slightly to +1 sphere − 2.0 cyl axis 10°. Corneal topography 4 months after TA-LASIK showed marked improvement of the irregularity (**Figure 8.4**). Some residual with-the-rule (WTR) astigmatism was still present, but the irregular astigmatism which was present preoperatively had virtually disappeared as shown by the differential map (**Figure 8.4**).

## PATIENT ASJ: ASYMMETRIC WTR-ASTIGMATISM

This patient is an excellent example for the use of TA-LASIK in a cornea with "just" some asymmetric astigmatism. Remember, as many as 40 percent of human corneas show some asymmetries like the one shown here ! This 29-year-old lady had a refraction of –7 sphere –1.25 cyl axis 170° in her right eye. SCVA was 20/20. Corneal topography showed asymmetric WTR-astigmatism, with the lower half-meridian being steeper than the upper half-meridian (**Figure 8.5**, upper left). A symmetrical ablation pattern would have left part of the astigmatism in the lower half-meridian. We therefore decided to perform TA-LASIK

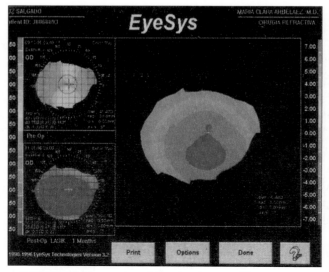

**FIGURE 8.5:** Pre- and postoperative topographic maps and differential map of patient ASJ (asymmetric WTR-astigmatism)

in this patient. Preoperative pachymetry was 579 m. An optical zone size of 5 mm was used. Flap thickness was 160 m, and ablation depth was 109 m.

On day 1, UCVA was 20/30 and BCVA (+1.25) was 20/20. At 1 month.

UCVA was 20/20, and results remained stable throughout the follow-up period of 6 months. Corneal topography showed a spherical surface after the ablation (**Figure 8.5**, lower left). The differential maps nicely demonstrates the asymmetric ablation performed— flattening was greater in the lower half-meridian than in the upper half-meridian, as clearly visible by the asymmetric blue bow-tie pattern (**Figure 8.5**).

## PATIENTS AND RESULTS

In a prospective, noncomparative case series, we operated 29 consecutive eyes of 27 patients between July 1996 and July 1997. All eyes have one year follow-up, and the data were presented at the annual meeting of the American Academy of Ophthalmology in New Orleans in 1998. Results were evaluated in four groups:

*Group 1* (post-keratoplasty group) consisted of six eyes (five patients) with irregular corneal astigmatism after penetrating keratoplasty. All grafts were performed more than 2 years ago.

*Group 2* (post-trauma group) consisted of six eyes (six patients) with irregular corneal astigmatism after corneal trauma. The trauma dated back more than 2 years in all eyes.

*Group 3* (decentered/small optical zones group) consisted of 11 eyes (10 patients) with irregular corneal astigmatism after PRK (one eye) or LASIK (10 eyes) due to decentered or small optical zones. All patients complained about halos and image distortion even during the day.

*Group 4* (central islands group) consisted of six eyes (six patients) with irregular astigmatism after PRK (two eyes) or LASIK (four eyes) due to central islands or keyhole patterns. All patients complained about blurred vision or image distortion even during the day.

Corneal topography was performed using the corneal analysis system (EyeSys System 2000, Software Version 3.10 and 3.20, EyeSys Premier, Irvine, CA) and more recently the Technomed C-Scan (Technomed Co., Baesweiler, Germany). The topographic changes from the preoperative examination to the postoperative examination at 12 months were subjectively graded as follows—planned correction fully achieved (irregularity less than 1 D and optical zone size as predicted), attempted correction partially achieved (decrease of irregularity of more than 1 D on the differential map and/or increase of optical zone size by at least 1 mm), flattening or steepening of the corneal contour level only, no change of irregularity (change 1 D or less on differential map), no change at all. The term "topographic success rate" (see **Table 8.1**) was introduced and defined to include eyes in which the planned correction was fully achieved and eyes in which the planned correction was partially achieved. In addition, a short questionnaire was completed 12 months after surgery by all patients. Patients were asked to rate their satisfaction with the result of the surgery (high, moderate, not satisfied).

The results of all groups are given in **Table 8.1**. In the postkeratoplasty group, corrective cylinder was significantly reduced as compared to the preoperative value, and UCVA improved significantly. In the posttrauma group, corrective cylinder was also significantly reduced, and UCVA improved significantly. In the decentered/small optical zones group, both corrective cylinder and SE were reduced, and UCVA improved accordingly, but differences were not statistically significant.

In the central islands group, both corrective cylinder and SE were reduced, and UCVA improved accordingly, but the difference of corrective cylinders was statistically significant only.

Comparing the groups, UCVA improved most in the postkeratoplasty and the posttrauma groups. Results were worst in the central island group, with 33 percent loosing two or more lines of UCVA.

Results of corneal topography were best in the decentered/small optical zones group, with a success rate, defined as the percentage of eye with the planned result and the percentage of eyes that improved, of 91 percent, followed by the posttrauma group with a success rate of 83 percent. The lowest success rate was observed in the central island group, being 50 percent only (**Table 8.1**).

**Table 8.1:** Refraction, visual acuity, corneal topography, and patient satisfaction 12 months after topographically-guided LASIK

|  | Group 1 Postkeratoplasy | Group 2 Posttrauma | Group 3 Decentered/small | Group 4 Central islands |
|---|---|---|---|---|
| No. of eyes | n = 6 | n = 6 | n = 11 | n = 6 |
| Cylinder preoperatively | 5.83 +/- 1.25 D (4.00 to 8.00 D) | 2.21 +/- 1.35 D (1.00 to 5.00 D) | 0.73 +/- 0.71 D (0 to 2.00 D) | 1.42 +/- 1.13 D (0 to 3.50 D) |
| Cylinder at 12 months | 2.96 +/- 1.23 D* (1.50 to 4.50 D) | 0.50 +/- 0.84 D** (0 to 2.5 D) | 0.36 +/- 1.05 D (0 to 3.5 D) | 0.50 +/- 0.84 D* (0 to 2.00 D) |
| UCVA improved 2 or more lines | 83% | 83% | 55% | 50% |
| UCVA +/-1 line | 17% | 17% | 36% | 17% |
| UCVA lost 2 or more lines | 0% | 0% | 9% | 33% |
| Topographic success rate | 66% (n = 4) | 83% (n = 5) | 91% (n = 10) | 50% (n = 3) |
| Patient response: "Very satisfied" | 66% (n = 4) | 66% (n = 4) | 18% (n = 2) | 34% (n = 2) |
| Patient response: "Moderately satisfied" | 17% (n = 1) | 0% | 46% (n = 5) | 0% |
| Patient response: "Not satisfied" | 17% (n = 1) | 34% (n = 2) | 36% (n = 4) | 66% (n = 4) |
| Reoperation rate | 50% (n = 3) | 50% (n = 3) | 36% (n = 4) | 50% (n = 3) |

SE—spherical equivalent of manifest refraction, UCVA—uncorrected visual acuity, * p—0.01; ** p—0.001

## SUMMARY

We observed a significant improvement of UCVA, a significant reduction of corrective cylinder, and a more regular corneal topography in all but one of the treatment groups. However, results were poor in one group (central islands group). Our results confirm that topographically-guided LASIK works clinically, and that it is clearly indicated in decentered or small optical zones and useful in postkeratoplasty and posttrauma irregularities. Following refinement of targeting, ablation algorithms, and corneal topography systems, topographically-guided LASIK will in the near future be a tool to create hard-contact lens vision in patients with irregular or asymmetric corneas. Topography-assisted LASIK will take refractive surgery to new limits by ultimately providing a quality of vision which is better than ever before in those 40 percent of patients with corneal irregularities.

# Chapter 9

# *Aberropia: A New Refractive Entity*

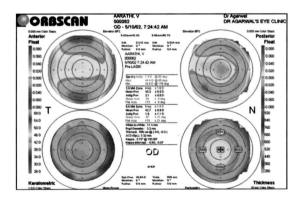

*Amar  Agarwal*
*Athiya  Agarwal*
*Sunita  Agarwal*

## INTRODUCTION

The next evolution to come on to the visual science scene in refractive ocular imaging is the aberrometer, the Orbscan and wave front analysis. This technology is based on astrophysical principles, which astronomers use to perfect the images impinging on their telescopes. Dr. Bille, the Director of the Institute of Applied Physics at the University of Heidelberg first began work in this field while developing this specific technology for astronomy applications in the mid-1970's. For perfect imaging, astrophysicists have to be able to measure and correct the imperfect higher-order aberrations or wavefront distortions that enter their telescopic lens system from the galaxy. To achieve this purpose, adaptive optics are used wherein deformable mirrors reform the distorted wavefront to allow clear visualization of celestial objects. Extrapolating these same principles to the human eye, it was thought that removal of the wavefront aberrations of the eye might finally yield the long awaited and much desired ultimate goal of "super vision".

So far, the only parameters that could be modified to obtain the optical correction for a given patient refractive error was the sphere, cylinder and axis even though this does not give the ideal optical correction many a times. This is because the current modes for correcting the optical aberrations of the eye do not reduce the higher order aberrations. The ideal optical system should be able to correct the optical aberrations in such a way that the spatial resolving ability of the eye is limited only by the limits imposed by the neural retina i.e. receptor diameter and receptor packing.

Thus, there may be a large group of patients whose best-corrected visual acuity (BCVA) may actually improve significantly on removal of the optical aberrations. These optical aberrations are contributed to by the eye's entire optical system i.e. the cornea, the lens, the vitreous and the retina. This study was conducted to determine the existence of a hitherto unidentified entity which we label as *"aberropia"* wherein patients with best-corrected visual acuity of £ 6/9 (0.63), corneal topography not accounting for the lack of improvement in BCVA and with no other known cause for decreased vision improved by ³ two Snellen lines after refractive correction of their wavefront aberration.

## MATERIALS AND METHODS

Sixteen eyes of ten patients were included in this retrospective study carried out at the Dr. Agarwal's Eye Institute, India between May to December 2002. Only patients who had visual acuity less than 6/9 (0.63) prior to the procedure and whose visual acuity improved by more than or equal to two lines after the procedure were included in the study. None of these patients had any other known cause for decreased vision and their corneal topography did not account for the lack of improvement in BCVA. The routine patient evaluation including uncorrected (UCVA) and best-corrected (BCVA), slit-lamp examination, applanation tonometry, manifest and cycloplegic refractions, Orbscan, aberrometry, corneal pachymetry, corneal diameter, Schirmer test and indirect ophthalmoscopy had been performed for all the patients. Patients wearing contact lenses had been asked to discontinue soft lenses for a minimum of 1 week and rigid gas permeable lenses for a minimum of 2 weeks before the preoperative examination and surgery. Informed consent was obtained form all patients after a thorough explanation of the procedure and its potential benefits and risks.

The Zyoptix procedure was then performed using the Bausch and Lomb Technolas 217 Z machine. The parameters used were: wavelength 193 nm, fluence 130 mJ/cm$^2$ and ablation zone diameters between 4.8mm and 6 mm. The Hansatome (Bausch and Lomb) was used in all the eyes. Either the 180 $\mu$m or the 160 $\mu$m plate was used in all the eyes. The aberrometer and the Orbscan, which checks the corneal topography, are linked and a zylink created. An appropriate software file is created which is then used to generate the laser treatment file.

Postoperatively, the patients underwent complete examination including UCVA, BCVA, slit lamp examination, Orbscan and aberrometry. The mean follow up was 37.5 days.

For statistical analysis, the Snellen acuity was converted to the decimal notation. Continuous variables were described with mean, standard deviation, minimum and maximum values.

## RESULTS

Sixteen eyes of ten patients satisfied the inclusion criteria. The mean age of the patients was 29.43 years (range 22 to 35 years). Six patients were females and 4 were males. The mean preoperative pupil diameter measured on aberrometer was 4.69 mm and mean postoperative pupil diameter measured on aberrometer was 4.53 mm.

The mean pre-operative spherical equivalent was − 4.94 D (range −12.50 to −1.5 D). The mean spherical equivalent at 1 month post-operative period was −0.16 ± 0.68 D (range −1.0 to 1.5) . Mean preoperative sphere was −4.95 D (range-12.50 to −0.75 D) and the mean postoperative sphere was −0.13 ± 0.68 D (range-1 to 1.5) at 1 month. The mean preoperative cylinder was −1.34 D (range 0 to −3.50). The mean postoperative cylinder was −0.08 ± 0.24 D (range 0 to −0.75 D) at one month. Postoperatively, at the end of first month, 70% of the patients were within ± 0.5D and 90% were within ± 1D of emmetropia **(Figure 9.1)**. Preoperatively mean RMS (Root Mean Square) values **(Figure 9.2)** were: Z 200 Defocus −9.22, Z 221 Astigmatism 0.12, Z 220 Astigmatism 1.02, Z 311 Coma −0.041, Z 310 Coma −0.04, Z 331 Trefoil 0.23, Z 330 Trefoil 0.016, Z 400 Spherical aberration −0.054, Z 420 Secondary astigmatism 0.103, Z 421 Secondary astigmatism 0.029, Z 440 Quadrafoil −0.103, Z 441 Quadrafoil −0.021, Z 510 Secondary coma 0.025, Z 511 Secondary coma −0.015, Z 530 Secondary trefoil 0.0049, Z 531 Secondary trefoil

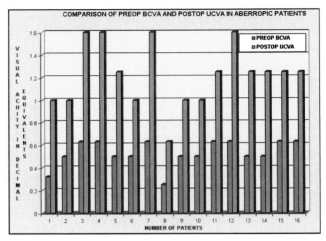

**FIGURE 9.1:** Pre-operative BCVA versus postoperative UCVA

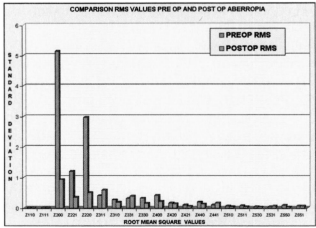

**FIGURE 9.2:** RMS values preoperative and postoperative

-0.00219, Z 550 Pentafoil 0.023, Z 551 Pentafoil 0.046. Postoperative mean RMS values were : Z 200 Defocus –0.429, Z 221 Astigmatism 0.07, Z 220 Astigmatism –0.07, Z 311 Coma 0.149, Z 310 Coma –0.079, Z 331 Trefoil –0.102, Z 330 Trefoil –0.004, Z 400 Spherical aberration -0.179, Z 420 Secondary astigmatism 0.015, Z 421 Secondary astigmatism 0.031, Z 440 Quadrafoil 0.019, Z 441 Quadrafoil –0.069, Z 510 Secondary coma –0.008, Z 511 Secondary coma 0.008, Z 530 Secondary Trefoil -0.002, Z 531 Secondary Trefoil –0.014, Z 550 Pentafoil 0.006, Z 551 Pentafoil 0.026.

RMS pre and post-laser showed a reduction in the higher order aberrations **(Tables 9.1 and 9.2)**. 6.25 percent patients achieved 6/9, 31.25% patients achieved [3] 6/6 (1.00), 37.50 percent achieved a BCVA of 6/5 (1.25) and 25 percent achieved a BCVA of 6/4 (1.6) **(Figure 9.3)**. **Figure 9.4** shows the pre-op Orbscan picture of a patient showing no abnormality. **Figures 9.5 and 9.6** show the aberrometer maps of the right eye and left eye of a patient in which we can see the aberrations reduced post laser.

## DISCUSSION

Zyoptix is the new generation of excimer laser used for the treatment of refractive disorders. Until recently, refractive disorders were treated with standard techniques, which took into consideration only the subjective refraction. Zyoptix technique on the other hand, takes into account the patient's subjective refraction, ocular

Table 9.1: RMS value pre-laser

| Patient No | Z110 | Z111 | Z200 | Z221 | Z220 | Z311 | Z310 | Z331 | Z330 | Z400 | Z420 | Z421 | Z440 | Z441 | Z510 | Z511 | Z530 | Z531 | Z550 | Z551 | Z6 |
|---|---|---|---|---|---|---|---|---|---|---|---|---|---|---|---|---|---|---|---|---|---|
| 1 | 0 | 0 | -5.77 | 4.055. | -6.131 | 0.299 | -0.113 | 0.725 | -0.44 | 0.009 | -0.03 | 0.102 | -0.233 | 0.109 | 0.131 | 0.027 | -0.048 | -0.041 | 0.052 | 0.039 | .9999 |
| 2 | 0 | 0 | -4.323 | -1.719 | 6.005 | -0.273 | 0.022 | -0.353 | 0.275 | 0.092 | 0.092 | -0.145 | 0.199 | -0.013 | -0.006 | 0.011 | 0.034 | -0.039 | 0.042 | 0.042 | .9999 |
| 3 | 0 | 0 | -11.8 | -0.088 | 0.116 | 0.435 | -0.658 | -0.444 | -0.567 | -0.779 | -0.089 | 0.043 | -0.202 | -0.053 | -0.052 | -0.057 | -0.04 | -0.001 | 0.13 | 0.111 | .9999 |
| 4 | 0 | 0 | -12.46 | 0.514 | -0.155 | 0.29 | -0.006 | 0.016 | 0.529 | -0.91 | 0.124 | 0.124 | -0.431 | -0.222 | 0.074 | -0.04 | 0.001 | -0.063 | -0.141 | 0.119 | .9999 |
| 5 | 0 | 0 | -6.535 | -0.123 | -0.886 | 0.156 | -0.09 | 0.094 | -0.128 | -0.084 | -0.072 | 0.035 | -0.009 | -0.044 | 0.001 | -0.031 | 0.01 | -0.005 | 0.001 | -0.041 | .9999 |
| 6 | 0 | 0 | -7.867 | 0.185 | 1.704 | -0.02 | 0.414 | 0.441 | 0.197 | 0.365 | 0.197 | 0.107 | -0.155 | -0.002 | 0.123 | 0.026 | -0.001 | 0.049 | 0.048 | 0.032 | .9999 |
| 7 | 0 | 0 | -4.28 | 0.167 | 2.571 | 0.007 | -0.089 | 0.356 | 0.125 | 0.585 | 0.101 | -0.002 | -0.17 | -0.062 | -0.077 | 0.198 | 0.001 | -0.104 | -0.022 | 0.029 | .9999 |
| 8 | 0 | 0 | -10.4 | 0.502 | -0.587 | -0.007 | -0.331 | 0.165 | -0.126 | -0.054 | -0.071 | 0.036 | -0.118 | -0.128 | 0.009 | 0.017 | -0.007 | -0.026 | 0.063 | -0.052 | .9999 |
| 9 | 0 | 0 | -17.15 | -0.414 | -1.217 | 0.093 | -0.106 | 0.343 | -0.18 | -0.254 | 0.009 | 0.002 | 0.001 | -0.025 | 0.007 | -0.022 | -0.007 | -0.042 | 0.037 | 0.04 | .9999 |
| 10 | 0 | 0 | -16.78 | -0.162 | -0.637 | 0.122 | -0.159 | 0.279 | 0.2 | -0.181 | 0.115 | 0.007 | -0.002 | 0.042 | -0.034 | -0.028 | 0.021 | -0.043 | -0.006 | -0.017 | .9999 |
| 11 | 0 | 0 | -4.513 | 2.916 | 4.661 | -0.634 | -0.205 | 0.477 | 0.44 | 0.094 | 0.377 | 0.058 | -0.201 | 0.101 | 0.133 | -0.147 | 0.009 | 0.011 | -0.055 | 0.118 | .9999 |
| 12 | 0 | 0 | -5.736 | -1.501 | 5.195 | -1.126 | 0.32 | 0.665 | -0.254 | 0.218 | 0.479 | 0.122 | -0.253 | -0.045 | 0.099 | -0.025 | 0.012 | -0.006 | -0.05 | 0.11 | .9999 |
| 13 | 0 | 0 | -15.46 | 1.605 | 2.754 | 0.378 | 0.443 | 0.208 | 0.458 | 0.643 | -0.083 | 0.09 | 0.407 | -0.006 | -0.021 | 0.09 | 0.033 | 0.032 | 0.239 | 0.149 | .9999 |
| 14 | 0 | 0 | -15.26 | -0.557 | 2.865 | -0.26 | -0.059 | 0.107 | 0.122 | 0.168 | 0.025 | -0.256 | -0.003 | 0.257 | 0.007 | 0.051 | 0.136 | -0.061 | -0.114 | 0.124 | .9999 |
| 15 | 0 | 0 | -4.955 | 0.735 | 0.383 | -0.401 | 0.003 | 0.62 | -0.494 | -0.676 | 0.391 | 0.163 | -0.421 | -0.264 | 0.039 | -0.261 | -0.079 | 0.241 | 0.103 | -0.067 | .9999 |
| 16 | 0 | 0 | -4.367 | -0.195 | -0.238 | 0.28 | -0.04 | 0.021 | 0.11 | -0.112 | 0.084 | -0.022 | -0.061 | 0.013 | -0.018 | -0.063 | 0.004 | 0.063 | 0.044 | 0 | .9999 |

**Table 9.2:** RMS value post-laser

| Pat No. | Z 110 | Z 111 | Z 200 | Z 221 | Z 220 | Z 311 | Z 310 | Z 331 | Z 330 | Z 400 | Z 420 | Z 421 | Z 440 | Z 441 | Z 510 | Z 511 | Z 530 | Z 531 | Z 550 | Z 551 | Z 6 |
|---|---|---|---|---|---|---|---|---|---|---|---|---|---|---|---|---|---|---|---|---|---|
| 1 | 0 | 0 | -0.022 | 0.74 | -1.294 | 0.117 | -0.067 | 0.141 | 0.052 | -0.063 | -0.076 | 0.1 | 0.054 | -0.037 | -0.028 | 0.001 | 0.008 | 0.007 | 0.013 | 0.006 | .9999 |
| 2 | 0 | 0 | -0.508 | 0.12 | 0.194 | -0.085 | 0.039 | -0.12 | -0.018 | .9999 | .9999 | .9999 | .9999 | .9999 | .9999 | .9999 | .9999 | .9999 | .9999 | .9999 | .9999 |
| 3 | 0 | 0 | -1.398 | -0.606 | 0.697 | -0.558 | -0.351 | 0.841 | 0.345 | -0.39 | 0.392 | 0.038 | -0.303 | -0.038 | -0.001 | 0.103 | -0.066 | -0.105 | -0.021 | 0.137 | .9999 |
| 4 | 0 | 0 | -2.05 | -0.499 | -0.375 | -0.027 | -0.269 | -0.534 | -0.289 | -0.58 | 0.114 | 0.058 | 0.236 | -0.161 | 0.034 | -0.083 | 0.004 | 0.039 | 0.01 | -0.077 | .9999 |
| 5 | 0 | 0 | 0.229 | 0.1 | -0.123 | -.9999 | -.9999 | -.9999 | -.9999 | -.9999 | -.9999 | -.9999 | -.9999 | -.9999 | -.9999 | -.9999 | -.9999 | -.9999 | -.9999 | -.9999 | .9999 |
| 6 | 0 | 0 | -0.036 | -0.17 | 0.425 | -0.002 | 0.069 | -0.045 | -0.042 | -0.342 | -0.032 | 0.094 | 0.075 | -0.05 | 0.068 | 0.03 | 0.064 | -0.014 | 0.012 | 0.002 | .9999 |
| 7 | 0 | 0 | 0.687 | 0.128 | -0.028 | -0.117 | -0.043 | 0.062 | 0.088 | -0.178 | 0.179 | 0.024 | -0.045 | 0.055 | 0.013 | 0.016 | -0.034 | -0.013 | -0.013 | 0.059 | .9999 |
| 8 | 0 | 0 | -2.164 | 0.279 | -0.696 | -0.25 | -0.398 | -0.147 | -0.128 | -0.581 | -0.238 | 0.02 | 0.032 | -0.088 | -0.129 | 0.028 | -0.029 | 0.007 | 0.089 | 0.059 | .9999 |
| 9 | 0 | 0 | -0.298 | 0.002 | -0.311 | 0.158 | -0.206 | 0.129 | -0.116 | -0.105 | -0.045 | -0.043 | 0.032 | -0.1 | .9999 | .9999 | .9999 | .9999 | .9999 | .9999 | .9999 |
| 10 | 0 | 0 | 0.109 | 0.241 | -0.503 | 0.233 | -0.119 | -0.16 | -0.204 | -.9999 | -.9999 | -.9999 | -.9999 | -.9999 | -.9999 | -.9999 | -.9999 | -.9999 | -.9999 | -.9999 | .9999 |
| 11 | 0 | 0 | 0.034 | -0.092 | 0.076 | 0.013 | -0.03 | -0.067 | 0.003 | -.9999 | -.9999 | -.9999 | -.9999 | -.9999 | -.9999 | -.9999 | -.9999 | -.9999 | -.9999 | -.9999 | .9999 |
| 12 | 0 | 0 | 0.187 | 0.061 | 0.004 | -0.097 | 0.015 | 0.067 | 0.035 | -.9999 | -.9999 | -.9999 | -.9999 | -.9999 | -.9999 | -.9999 | -.9999 | -.9999 | -.9999 | -.9999 | .9999 |
| 13 | 0 | 0 | -0.701 | 0.291 | 0.598 | 2.161 | 0.349 | -1.062 | -0.201 | -0.428 | -0.013 | 0.204 | 0.258 | -0.636 | -0.082 | 0.113 | 0.069 | -0.239 | 0.062 | .9999 | .9999 |
| 14 | 0 | 0 | -0.638 | 0.094 | 0.391 | 0.517 | -0.328 | -0.336 | 0.188 | -0.118 | -0.077 | 0.003 | 0.157 | 0.034 | -0.006 | -0.025 | 0.004 | 0.018 | -0.066 | .9999 | .9999 |
| 15 | 0 | 0 | -0.148 | 0.493 | 0.017 | 0.261 | 0.017 | -0.354 | 0.302 | -0.111 | 0.053 | 0.07 | -0.019 | -0.084 | -0.007 | -0.051 | -0.052 | 0.063 | 0.011 | .9999 | .9999 |
| 16 | 0 | 0 | -0.161 | -0.038 | -0.331 | 0.072 | 0.049 | -0.05 | -0.086 | 0.025 | -0.008 | -0.059 | -0.028 | -.9999 | -.9999 | -.9999 | -.9999 | -.9999 | -.9999 | -.9999 | .9999 |

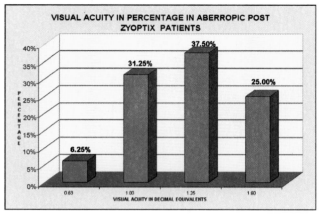

**FIGURE 9.3:** Percentage values of visual acuity

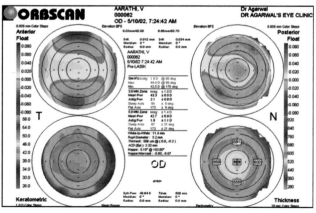

**FIGURE 9.4:** Pre-operative orbscan

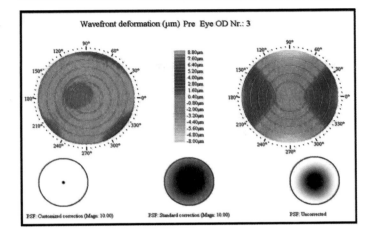

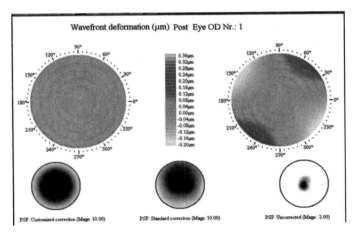

**FIGURE 9.5:** Pre and postoperative aberrometer maps of a patient showing removal of aberrations

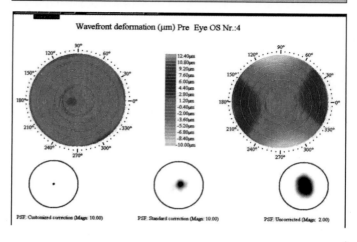

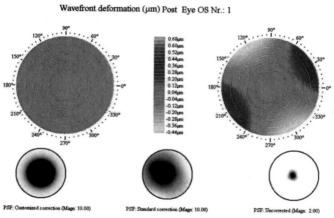

**FIGURE 9.6:** Pre and post-operative aberrometry of a patient showing removal of higher order aberrations

optical aberrations and corneal topography, with the latter not only for the diagnosis, but also for the therapeutic treatment, in order to design a personalized treatment based on the total structure of the eye. The wavefront technology in Zyoptix uses the Hartmann Shack aberrometer based on the Hartmann-Shack principle[1] demonstrated by Liang et al[2] to measure the eye's wave aberration. This wavefront sensor has been improved by increasing the density of samples taken of the wave-front slope in the pupil[3]. All Hartmann-Shack devices are outgoing testing devices in that they evaluate the light being bounced back out through the optical system. A narrow laser beam is focused onto the retina to generate a point source. The out coming light rays which experience all the aberrations of the eye pass through an array of lenses which detects their deviation. The wavefront deformation is calculated by analyzing the direction of the light rays using this lenslet array. Parallel light beams indicate a good wavefront and non-parallel light beams indicate a wavefront with aberrations, which does not give equidistant focal points. This image is then captured onto a ccd camera and the wavefront is reconstructed. The data is explained mathematically in three dimensions with polynomial functions. Most investigators have chosen the Zernike method for this analysis although Taylor series can also be used for the same purpose[4]. Data from the wavefront map is presented as a sum of Zernike polynomials each describing a certain deformation. At any point in the pupil, the wavefront aberration is the optical path difference between the actual image wavefront and the ideal spherical wavefront centered at the image point[5].

Any refractive error which cannot be corrected by sphero-cylindrical lens combinations is referred to by physicists as higher order aberrations i.e., comma, spherical aberration, chromatic aberration. The Zernike Polynomials, which describe ray points, are used to obtain a best fit toric to correct for the refractive error of the eye. The points are described in the x and y coordinates and the third dimension, height, is described in the z-axis. The local refractive correction of each area of the entrance pupil can be determined by calculating from the wavefront polynomial the corresponding local radii of curvature and hence the required spherocylindrical correction[6]. Thus, each small region of the entrance pupil has its own three parameters that characterize the local refractive correction: sphere, cylinder and axis[6]. The global aberrations of the entire optical system including the cornea, lens, vitreous and the retina are thus measured. The great advantage of wavefront analysis is that it can describe these other aberrations.

The first order polynomial describes the spherical error or power of the eye. The second order polynomial describes the regular astigmatic component and its orientation or axis. Third order aberrations are considered to be coma and fourth order aberrations are considered to be spherical aberration. Zernike polynomial descriptions for wavefront analysis typically go up to the tenth order of expression. The first and second orders describe the morphology of a normal straight curve. More local maximum and minimum points require higher orders of the polynomial series to describe the surface. Normal eyes exhibit spherical[7,8] and coma[9,10] aberrations in addition to exhibiting defocus and astigmatism.

Ideally, the difference in the magnitude of the local refractive correction of each area of the entrance pupil should not exceed 0.25 D. Lower spherocylindrical corrections are generally associated with lower wavefront aberrations.[6] These observations regarding variation in local ocular refraction along different meridians are also confirmed by Ivanoff[11] and Jenkins.[12] Van den Brink[13] also commented on the change in refraction across the pupil. Clinically significant changes of at least 0.25 D in one or both components of the spherocylindrical correction might normally be expected for decentrations of about 1 mm. Rayleigh's quarter wavelength rule states that if the wavefront aberration exceeds a quarter of a wavelength, the quality of the retinal image will be impaired significantly.[14] Thus the aberration in eyes starts to become significant when the pupil diameter exceeds 1-2 mm[6]. Thus it is not possible to correct the entire wavefront aberration with a single spherocylindrical lens. As conventional refractive procedures such as LASIK also reduce only the second order aberrations, the visual acuity will still be limited by aberrations of third and higher order aberrations. These patients are likely to undergo tremendous improvement in their BCVA after correction of their aberrations by Zyoptix.

In the Zyoptix system, the aberrometer and the orbscan, which checks the corneal topography, are linked and a zylink created. An appropriate software file is created which is then used to generate the laser treatment file. The truncated gaussian beam shape used in Zyoptix combines the advantages of the common beam shapes, i.e. flat top beam and the gaussian beam, creating a maximized smoothness and minimized thermal effect. Thus Zyoptix gives a smoother corneal surface, reducing glare and increasing visual acuity. The larger optical zones reduce haloes. Zyoptix also causes a reduction of the ablation depth by 15 to 20 percent and a reduced enhancement rate.

In a patient with higher order aberrations, LASIK does not remove the higher order aberrations and the point-spread function is a large blur. Zyoptix on the other hand, performs customized ablation and removes the higher order aberrations thus minimizing the wavefront deformation. The point-spread function is therefore a small spot of light.

In our study, the mean preoperative spherical equivalent improved from –4.78 D to –0.16 D ± 0.68 and the mean preoperative cylinder improved from –1.34 D to –0.08 D ± 0.24. The aberrations were reduced drastically in all the eyes and the BCVA improved in all cases by ≤ two lines. Reduction of the aberrations of the eye can thus result in an improved BCVA postoperatively.

Improving the optics of the eye by removing aberrations increases the contrast and spatial detail of the retinal image. Reduction of higher order aberrations may not improve high contrast acuity much more in eyes where spherocylindrical lenses alone improve the BCVA to 6/3 (2.00) or better. In contrast, in otherwise normal eyes where the BCVA is limited to 6/9 (0.50) or 6/6 (1.00) due to optical aberrations, reduction of higher order aberrations should improve visual acuity.

Realization of the best possible unaided visual acuity may be limited at the cortical, retinal and the spectacle, corneal, or implant level. All maculae may not be able to support 6/3 (2.00) vision. Insufficient cone density or sub-optimal orientation of cone receptors or a sub-optimal Stiles-Crawford profile of the macula may make 6/3 (2.00) vision impossible. Clinical or sub-clinical amblyopia may make achievement of super vision impossible. But, in spite of this, there may be a certain patient population who have the potential for an improved BCVA on removal of their wavefront aberrations. The corneal topography does not account for the decreased preoperative visual acuity in these patients, neither do they have any other identifiable cause for the decrease in acuity except for an abnormal wavefront. It is important that this subgroup of patients are identified and their optical aberrations neutralized so that they are not deprived of the opportunity to gain in their BCVA.

Wavefront sensing technology, at present, does not in most cases define the exact locale of the pathology causing the aberration. Hence, clinical examination and other refractive tools, such as corneal topographic mapping, along with sound clinical judgment is required for proper understanding of the eye and its individual refractive status. Also, wavefront aberrations may not remain static. Numerous authors[15-18] have shown that ocular optical aberrations probably remain constant between 20 and 40 years of age but increase after that. Aberrations also change during accommodation [19,20] and may be affected by mydriatics.[21] Thus, the patient should be informed about these possibilities while taking the consent for the procedure. Long term studies are required to determine the stability of the post-operative refraction, residual aberrations and changes in BCVA if any.

The question of magnification factor improving visual acuity does not arise as these patients pre-operatively did not improve with contact lenses. Further the refractive error in some of these patients was not very large.

## CONCLUSION

In conclusion, removal of the wavefront aberration may extend the benefit of an improved BCVA to patients with an abnormal wavefront. The subgroup of patients with higher order aberrations, normal corneal topography and no other known cause for decreased vision may thus benefit immensely with wavefront guided refractive surgery. Customized refractive surgery tailor-made for these individual patients, aimed at neutralizing the wavefront aberrations of the eye is safer, more predictable, provides better visual acuities and reduces the incidence of unsatisfactory outcomes. Further studies are required to assess the long-term outcomes.

Till now, when we discuss refractive errors we discuss about spherical and a cylindrical correction. But in todays world we have to think of a third parameter which is the aberrations present in the eye which can be anywhere in the optical media. These can be corrected in the corneal level by the laser treatment.

## REFERENCES

1. B Platt, RV Shack. Lenticular Hartmann screen. Opt Sci Center News (University of Arizona) 1971;5:15-16.
2. J Liang, B Grimm, S Goelz, J Bille. Objective measurement of the wave aberrations of the human eye with the use of a Hartmann-Shack wavefront sensor. J Opt Soc Am 1994; 11: 1949-57.
3. J Liang, D R Williams et al. Aberrations and retinal image quality of the normal human eye. J Opt Soc Am A 1997; 14(11): 2873-83.
4. Oshika T, Klyce SD, Applegate RA et al. Comparison of corneal wavefront aberrations after photorefractive keratectomy and laser in situ keratomileusis. Am J Ophthalmol 1999; 127:1-7.
5. Fincham WHA, Freeman MH. Optics. 9th ed. London: Butterworths, 1980. Born M, Wolf E. Principles of Optics. 2nd edn. New York: Macmillan, 1964:203-32.
6. WN Charman, G Walsh. Variations in the local refractive correction of the eye across its entrance pupil. Optometry and Vision Science 1989;66(1):34-40.
7. WM Rosenblum and JL Christensen. Objective and subjective spherical aberration measurement of the human eye. In Wolf E (Ed): Progress in Optics. North-Holland, Amsterdam, 1976;13:69-91
8. MC Campbell, EM Harrison, P Simonet. Psychophysical measurement of the blur on the retina due to optical aberrations of the eye. Vision Res 1990; 30:1587-1602.
9. HC Howland, B Howland. A subjective method for the measurement of monochromatic aberrations of the eye. J Opt Soc Am 1977; 67: 1508-18.

10. G Walsh, WN Charman, HC Howland. Objective technique for the determination of monochromatic aberrations of the human eye. J Opt Soc Am A 1984; 1:987-992.

11. Ivanoff A. About the spherical aberration of the eye. J Opt Soc Am 1956;46: 901-03.

12. Jenkins TCA. Aberrations of the eye and their effects on vision. Part 1. Br J Physiol Opt 1963; 20: 59-91.

13. Van den Brink G. Measurements of the geometric aberrations of the eye. Vision Res. 1962; 2: 233-44.

14. Born M, Wolf E. Principles of Optics. 2nd ed. New York: Macmillan 1964;203-32.

15. Kaemmerer M, Mrochen M, Mierdel p, et al. Optical aberrations of the human eye. Nature Medicine (in press).

16. Oshika T, Klyce SD, Applegate RA, et al. Changes in corneal wavefront aberration with aging. Invest Ophthalmol Vis Sci 1999; 40: 1351-55.

17. Calver RI, Cox MJ, Elliot DB. Effect of aging on the monochromatic aberrations of the human eye. J Opt Soc Am A 1999; 16: 2069-2078.

18. Guirao A, Gonzalez C, Redondo M et al. Average optical performance of the human eye as a function of age in a normal population. Invest Ophthalmol Vis Sci 1999; 40 203-13.

19. Krueger R, Kaemerrer M, Mrochen M et al. Understanding refraction and accommodation through "ingoing optics" aberrometry: a case report. Ophthalmology (in press).

20. He JC, Burns SA, Marcos S. Monochromatic aberrations in the accommodated human eye. Vis Res 2000; 40:41-48.

21. Fankhauser F, Kaemerrer M, Mrochen M et al. The effect of accommodation, mydriasis, and cycloplegia on aberrometry. ARVO abstract 2248. Invest Ophthalmol Vis Sci 2000; 41; S461.

# Chapter 10

# *Topographic and Pachymetric Changes Induced by Contact Lenses*

*Melania Cigales*
*Jairo E Hoyos*
*Jorge Pradas*

## INTRODUCTION

Hartstein[1] was the first to note contact lens-induced changes in corneal shape and to refer to them as *corneal warpage*.

More recent publications[2] define the term corneal warpage as denoting all contact lens-induced changes in corneal topography, reversible or permanent, that are not associated with corneal edema.

Patients with contact lens-induced corneal warpage are commonly asymptomatic.[3] These patients frequently do not use glasses and depend on their contact lenses for their refractive error. Some may also notice intolerance to contact lenses or decreased visual acuity with glasses.

Reported signs of contact lens-induced corneal warpage[1,4-7] include changes in refraction and keratometric readings (relative steepening of mean corneal curvature in some patients, and flattening in others) and distortion of keratometer or keratoscope mires. But the keratometer evaluates corneal curvature from only four paracentral points, approximately 3 mm apart. The keratoscope provides information from a larger portion of the corneal surface, but the data are qualitative in nature. For these reasons, the best system to study contact lens-induced corneal warpage is computer-assisted topographic analysis of videokeratoscopic images.[8]

Contact lens-induced topographical abnormalities of the cornea include
- Central irregular astigmatism
- Loss of radial symmetry

- Reversal of the normal topographic pattern of progressive flattening of corneal contour from the center to the periphery
- Keratoconus-like images.[2,3,9-12]

Some studies[13,14] show corneal thickness modifications induced by contact lens wear. There have been reports of increased corneal thickness measured by an optical pachymeter which have shown that this finding is mainly due to oxygen deprivation leading to corneal edema. Other researchers[15] have found, in histopathological studies, that there is a reduced corneal thickness resulting from epithelial thinning. We have not found reports of studies done with the use of ultrasound pachymetry.

## REFRACTIVE SURGERY IN CONTACT LENS WEARERS

Laser-assisted *"in-situ"* keratomileusis (LASIK) is a refractive surgery technique in which an attempt is made to correct ametropia by modifying the anterior surface of the cornea. Contact lens wear may induce transient modifications on the corneal surface, with refractive changes that have a negative impact on the predictability of the procedure.

In some cases, contact lenses may even produce corneal thinning, requiring the surgeon to program a smaller optic zone in order to correct the ametropia to avoid removing too much tissue. Hence, the importance of knowing the length of time, such patients should discontinue the use of contact lenses before undergoing surgery, as well as the parameters that might allow us to suspect corneal warpage derived from contact lens wear.

Studies have demonstrated that topographic alterations are common in normal wearers of soft and rigid gas-permeable (RGP) contact lenses. It is important to identify such topographic abnormalities before surgery, because they are likely to have an adverse effect on predictability and other determinants of the efficacy of refractive surgical procedures. Patients with contact lenses are required to discontinue their use before refractive surgery. Some authors[16] recommend 1 week for soft lenses and 2 weeks for RGP lenses, while others[17] recommend 2 weeks for all types of contact lenses.

It is our routine practice to discontinue contact lens wear before refractive surgery, 1 or 2 weeks for soft lenses and 1 month for RGP lenses. Despite this practice, we have found topographic patterns of corneal warpage in 22 eyes of 12 patients, 13 eyes with RGP lenses, and 9 eyes with soft lenses, followed every 2 to 4 weeks. At each visit, these patients were checked by topography, cycloplegic refraction, visual acuity and ultrasound pachymetry. Follow-up was continued until a topographic pattern, normal or abnormal, was found to persist without changes for at least 1 month.[3]

All eyes returned to their normal topographic pattern, except for one RGP lens wearer, who improved substantially and stabilized at 8 weeks, but never returned to a normal pattern. The mean time required for returning to a normal (or abnormal but stable), topographic pattern was 9 weeks (range from 4 to 10) for soft contact lens wearers, and 11 weeks (range from 8 to 16) for RGP contact lens wearers. These results are comparable to those obtained by Wilson et al.[3]

Before refractive surgery, RGP contact lenses must definitely be discontinued for a longer period of time than soft contact lenses. A period of 1 or 2 weeks for soft lenses and 1 month for RGP lenses may be appropriate, but if there are any topographical signs of corneal warpage, patients must be delayed until their patterns normalize and/or stabilize.

## PARAMETRIC DESCRIPTORS OF CORNEAL TOPOGRAPHY

Topographic analysis is the most sensitive method to detect subclinical or occult corneal warping, and as such should be the indicator for the time during which contact lens wear must be discontinued before refractive surgery.

In our study, we used a computerized topographic analysis with the TMS-1 topographer (Computed Anatomy Inc, software release 1.61, New York, NY). This instrument includes 25 videokeratoscopic rings covering almost the entire corneal surface, and digitizes 256 points along each mire. The international scale color code mapping was used to monitor corneal topography. Three topographic parameters were analyzed for follow-up: (i) *simulated keratoscope reading* (Sim K), (ii) *surface asymmetry index* (SAI), and (iii) *surface regularity index* (SRI).[3,10,18]

## SIMULATED KERATOSCOPE READING (SIM K)

The Sim K is calculated from the maximum meridian powers of rings, 6, 7 and 8. The display includes the average of those maximum powers, the axis at which the average value occurs, and the average power of the corneal surface for the same rings at the meridian located 90° away. Clinically insignificant cylindrical readings lower than 0.20 diopters (D) are not reported; instead, the spherical equivalent is reported in those cases. Sim K is used to quantify the dioptric power of the cornea in order to calculate the value of the cylinder and of the topographic axis, thus identifying differences between the initial and final examinations.[18]

## SURFACE ASYMMETRY INDEX (SAI)

The SAI is the centrally weighted sum of the differences in corneal power between corresponding points on the TMS-1 mires located 180° apart. The power distribution across a normal corneal surface is highly symmetrical, making the SAI a useful quantitative indicator for monitoring changes in corneal topography. Normal corneas generally have SAI values lower than 0.5. The SAI is correlated with potential visual acuity (PVA) as originally described by Klyce and Wilson, and is, to our knowledge, the first attempt at correlating the optical quality of corneal surfaces to visual acuity.[2,3]

## SURFACE REGULARITY INDEX (SRI)

The SRI is a quantitative descriptor which, like SAI, attempts to correlate the optical quality of the corneal surface with

PVA. The SRI is calculated on the basis of the local regularity of the surface over the corneal area enclosed by an average virtual pupil of approximately 4.5 mm. Like SAI, the SRI of normal corneal surfaces is relatively low, and higher SRI values indicate surface of lesser optical quality.[2,3]

## SOFT LENS-INDUCED CORNEAL CHANGES

Our results were consistent with those of previous studies[3,10,11] showing that soft contact lens-induced corneal warpage determines a topographic pattern of corneal steepening and increased myopia.

Changes occurring between the first and the last examinations revealed a reduction of myopia in 88.9 percent of the eyes, with an average of –2.11 D (range from –1 to – 6), associated with an average topographic flattening of 1.64 D (range from 0.05 to 4.15). These changes proved to be statistically significant and there was a positive correlation between them ($p<0.05$). The greater changes were found in cases of corneal warpage with keratoconus-like images.

**Figures 10.1A and B** show a clinical case of corneal warpage in a soft contact lens wear, with typical topographic pattern. **Figures 10.2A and B** show a clinical case of soft contact lens-induced corneal warpage, with keratoconus-like image.

Our study did not reveal changes in average astigmatic values after discontinuing contact lens wear.

| | 10 days without CL | 5 weeks without CL |
|---|---|---|
| Refraction | -16 -3 x 180º | -13 -1 x 180º |
| BCVA | 20/60 | 20/25 |
| Sim K | 46.5 x 44.5 | 43.2 x 42.1 |
| SAI | 0.77 | 0.21 |
| SRI | 1.11 | 0.44 |
| Pachymetry | 510 microns | 530 microns |

***FIGURE 10.1A*** (Case study 1): Soft contact lens-induced corneal warpage. Forty-eight-year-old female, permanent soft contact lens (CL) wearer for 2 years (removes them every 6 months for cleaning)

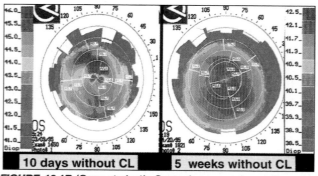

| 10 days without CL | 5 weeks without CL |

***FIGURE 10.1B*** (Case study 1): Corneal warpage in a soft contact lens wear with typical topographic pattern

However, these values were found to be reduced in 55.5 percent of cases, increased in 44.5 percent, and with axis modifications of more than 20° in 22.2 percent of cases.

Visual acuity improved from one to five Snellen lines in 66.7 percent of cases, coinciding with improved regularity and radial symmetry in the topographic image

|  | 10 days without CL | 5 weeks without CL |
|---|---|---|
| Refraction | -32 -1 x 10º | -25 |
| BCVA | 20/50 | 20/40 |
| Sim K | 47.8 x 46.5 | 43.3 x 42.7 |
| SAI | 0.64 | 0.22 |
| SRI | 1.09 | 0.22 |
| Pachymetry | 494 microns | 520 microns |

*FIGURE 10.2A* (Case study 2): Soft contact lens-induced corneal warpage. Thirty-eight-year-old male, soft contact lens (CL) wearer for 20 years, 16 to 18 hours/day

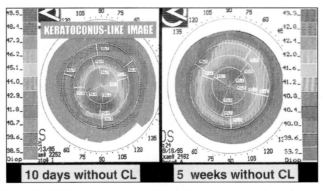

*FIGURE 10.2B* (Case study 2): Corneal warpage in a soft contact lens wear with keratoconus-like image in the topography

(SAI and SRI decreased in 90% and 100% of cases, respectively, reaching a final value $\leq 0.5$ in all cases). Improvements in visual acuity, and their relationship with symmetry (SAI) and regularity (SRI) indices have been described by other authors.[3,8,10,16,18]

Central corneal thickness was followed with ultrasound pachymetry (DGH-500 pachymeter, DGH Technology, Inc USA), revealing an increase in corneal thickness after discontinuation of soft contact lens wear in 90 percent of cases. The average increase in thickness was 20 microns (range from 0 to 30) and was statistically significant ($p < 0.05$). Wilson and Klyce[3,9,11] have associated this corneal thinning with the presence of keratoconus, but our results show topographic and pachymetric reversibility once contact lens wear is discontinued, ruling out the presence of keratoconus in those cases. In only one case did we diagnose keratoconus on the basis of persistent topographic alterations and corneal thinning, and this case was excluded from the study.

**To summarize, soft contact lenses may induce corneal warpage with topographic steepening (with an occasional keratoconus-like image) and increased myopia, as well as central corneal thinning. If all factors are not taken into consideration before refractive surgery, the result will be overcorrection and the selection of a smaller optic zone.**

## RGP LENS-INDUCED CORNEAL CHANGES

Our results show that RGP contact lens-induced corneal warpage is reflected in a topographic pattern of central corneal flattening and decreased myopia, and in cases of contact lens decentering, there is a keratoconus-like image. These results are consistent with the findings of other reported studies.[2,3,10-12]

Changes occurring between the first and the last examination revealed an increase in myopia in 77 percent of eyes, with an average of $-0.53$ D (range from $+1$ to $-1.12$), associated with an average topographic steepening of 0.43 D (range from 0.15 to 0.95). These changes proved to be statistically significant, and there was a positive correlation between them ($p < 0.05$). In this group, there were a few cases of relative topographic flattening with increased myopia after discontinuing RGP lens use. This coincided with decentered lenses, causing a flattening at the site of contact with the cornea and steepening on the other side, giving rise to a keratoconus-like image.[3]

**Figures 10.3A and B** show a clinical case of corneal warpage in a RGP contact lens wear, with typical topographic pattern. **Figures 10.4A and B** show a clinical case of RGP lens-induced corneal warpage, with keratoconus-like image.

Our study did not reveal changes in average astigmatic values after discontinuing contact lens wear. However, these values were found to be reduced in 18.2 percent of cases and increased in 18.2 percent, and there were axis modifications of more than $20°$ in 27.3 percent of cases.

In our study, we have found greater cylinder changes when soft contact lenses are discontinued (reduction in 55.5% and increase in 18.2% of cases) than the ones found in RGP lens wearers (reduction in 18.2% and increase in 18.2% of cases). Wilson and Klyce[3] report that astigmatic modifications are greater in RGP lens wearers in terms of a cylinder increase when lens wear is

|  | 4 weeks without CL | 9 weeks without CL |
|---|---|---|
| Refraction | -9.5 -1.5 x 10° | -11 -0.75 x 20° |
| BCVA | 20/30 | 20/20 |
| Sim K | 41.2 x 39.4 | 41.6 x 40.8 |
| SAI | 0.45 | 0.23 |
| SRI | 0.34 | 0.33 |
| Pachymetry | 480 microns | 505 microns |

**FIGURE 10.3A** (Case study 3): Rigid gas-permeable (RGP) contact lens-induced corneal warpage. Thirty-seven-year-old male, RGP contact lens (CL) wearer for 20 years, 16 to 18 hours/day

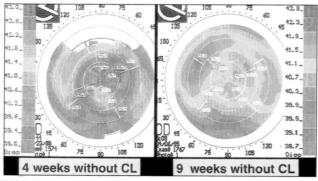

4 weeks without CL          9 weeks without CL

**FIGURE 10.3B** (Case study 3): Corneal warpage in a RGP contact lens wear with typical topographic pattern

discontinued, contrary to what happens with soft contact lenses.

There was an improvement of one to four Snellen lines of visual acuity in 38.5 percent of cases, coinciding with improved regularity and radial symmetry in the

|  | 1 week without CL | 12 weeks without CL |
|---|---|---|
| Refraction | -8.5 -1 x 40º | -7.5 -1 x 10º |
| BCVA | 20/30 | 20/25 |
| Sim K | 44.1 x 42.7 | 44.3 x 42.7 |
| SAI | 1.58 | 0.53 |
| SRI | 1.15 | 0.54 |
| Pachymetry | 543 microns | 555 microns |

*FIGURE 10.4A* (Case study 4): Rigid gas-permeable (RGP) contact lens-induced corneal warpage. Twenty-six-year-old female, RGP contact lens (CL) wearer for 10 years, 14 hours/day

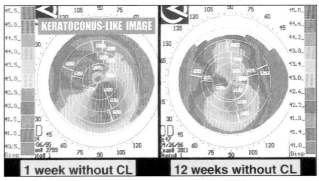

1 week without CL    12 weeks without CL

*FIGURE 10.4B* (Case study 4): Corneal warpage in a RGP contact lens wear with keratoconus-like image in the topography

topographic image (SAI and SRI decreased in 92% and 61.5% of cases, respectively, reaching a final value ≤ 0.5 in all cases). Improvements of visual acuity, and of symmetry and regularity indices, have been described by other authors.[2,3,8,10,16,18]

Follow-up on central corneal thickness with ultrasound pachymetry showed an increase in corneal thickness after RGP lenses were discontinued in 90 percent of cases, with an average increase of 15.5 microns (range from 0 to 25), which was statistically significant ($p < 0.05$). No differences were observed concerning pachymetric modifications in soft and RGP contact lens wearers.

To summarize, RGP contact lenses may induce corneal warpage with topographic flattening (with keratoconus-like images when decentered) and decreased myopia, as well as central corneal thinning. If all factors are not taken into consideration before refractive surgery, the result will be undercorrection and the selection of a smaller optic zone.

## CONCLUSION

It is essential to perform a critical evaluation of the corneal topography of all candidates prior to refractive surgery. The tendency to proceed immediately to surgery if the topography appears normal should be avoided because the initial topography may depart significantly from the one obtained before contact lens fitting.

Contact lens wear should be discontinued before refractive surgery for a period of 1 to 2 weeks for soft lenses, and 1 month for RGP lenses. However, in the event that any topographic signs of corneal warpage are observed, they must be followed until they normalize and/or stabilize. Therefore, topography will dictate the timing for refractive surgery.

The presence of topographic signs of corneal warpage must lead us to suspect the possibility of corneal thinning as a result of contact lens wear, requiring close topographic as well as pachymetric follow-up in these patients.

Careful operative evaluation and management are likely to improve the quality and predictability of corneal surgery of individual surgeons. Perhaps more importantly, the overall efficacy of procedures such as LASIK might be enhanced once unpredictable variables of contact lens-induced warpage are controlled.

## REFERENCES

1. Hartstein J. Corneal warping due to wearing of corneal contact lenses. Am J Ophthalmol 1965; 60: 1103-04.
2. Wilson SE, Lin DTC, Klyce SD et al. Rigid contact lens decentration—a risk factor for corneal warpage. CLAO J 1990; 16: 177-82.
3. Wilson SE, Lin DTC, Klyce SD et al. Topographic changes in contact lens-induced corneal warpage. Ophthalmology 1990; 97: 734-44.
4. Rengstorff RH. Corneal curvature and astigmatic changes subsequent to contact lens wear. J Am Optom Assoc 1965; 36: 996-1000.
5. Levenson DS. Changes in corneal curvature with long-term PMMA contact lens wear. CLAO J 1983; 9: 121-25.
6. Levenson DS, Berry CV. Findings on follow-up of corneal warpage patients. CLAO J 1983; 9: 126-29.
7. Koetting RA, Castellano CF, Keating MJ. PMMA lenses worn for twenty years. J Am Optom Assoc 1986; 57: 459-61.
8. Wilson SE, Klyce SD. Advances in the analysis of corneal topography. Surv Ophthalmol 1991; 35: 269-77.
9. Wilson SE, Lin DTC, Klyce SD. Corneal topography of keratoconus. Cornea 1991; 10: 2-8.

10. Ruiz-Montenegro J, Mafra CH, Wilson SE et al. Corneal topographic alterations in normal contact lens wearers. Ophthalmology 1993; 100: 128-34.

11. Wilson SE, Klyce SD. Screening for corneal topographic abnormalities before refractive surgery. Ophthalmology 1994; 101: 147-52.

12. Benavides J, Gutierrez AM. Estudio del sindrome de deformación corneal inducido por lentes de contacto en diez ojos. Arch Soc Am Oftal Optom 1994; 24: 19-22.

13. Miller D. Contact lens-induced corneal curvature and thickness changes. Arch Ophthal 1968; 80: 430-32.

14. Millodot M. Effect of hard contact lenses on corneal sensitivity and thickness. Acta Ophthalmologica 1975; 53: 576-84.

15. Bergmanson JPG. Histopathological analysis of the corneal epithelium after contact lens wear. J Am Optom Assoc 1987; 58: 812-18.

16. Gimbel HV. Effect of contact lens wear on photorefractive keratectomy. CLAO J 1993; 19: 217-21.

17. Pallikaris IG, Siganos DS. Excimer laser in situ keratomileusis and photorefractive keratectomy for correction of high myopia. J Refract Corneal Surg 1994; 10: 498-510.

18. Wilson SE, Klyce SD. Quantitative descriptors of corneal topography. Arch Ophthalmol 1991; 109: 349-53.

# Index

# READER SUGGESTIONS SHEET

*Please help us to improve the quality of our publications by completing and returning this sheet to us.*

Title/Author: **Dr Agarwals' Step by Step Corneal Topography by Sunita Agarwal, Athiya Agarwal, Amar Agarwal**

Your name and address:

E-mail address,

Phone and Fax:

How did you hear about this book? [please tick appropriate box (es)]

☐ Direct mail from publisher  ☐ Conference

☐ Bookshop  ☐ Book review

☐ Lecturer recommendation  ☐ Friends

☐ Other (please specify)  ☐ Website

**Type of purchase:** ☐ Direct purchase ☐ Bookshop ☐ Friends

Do you have any brief comments on the book?

**Please return this sheet to the name and address given below.**

# JAYPEE BROTHERS
## MEDICAL PUBLISHERS (P) LTD
EMCA House, 23/23B Ansari Road, Daryaganj
New Delhi 110 002, India